OX

Ox ~~Handbook of~~
**Pharmaceutical
Medicine**

Oxford Specialist Handbooks published and forthcoming

Oxford Specialist Handbook of

Pharmaceutical Medicine

Adrian Kilcoyne

Medical Director,
Sanofi Pasteur MSD Ltd,
Maidenhead, UK

Daniel O'Connor

Medical Assessor,
Medicines and Healthcare products
Regulatory Agency (MHRA),
London, UK

Phil Ambery

Director of Clinical Research,
GlaxoSmithKline R&D,
London, UK

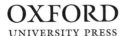

OXFORD
UNIVERSITY PRESS

OXFORD
UNIVERSITY PRESS

Great Clarendon Street, Oxford, OX2 6DP,
United Kingdom

Oxford University Press is a department of the University of Oxford.
It furthers the University's objective of excellence in research, scholarship,
and education by publishing worldwide. Oxford is a registered trade mark of
Oxford University Press in the UK and in certain other countries

British Library Cataloguing in Publication Data
Data available

ISBN 978–0–19–960914–7

Printed in China by
C&C Offset Printing Co. Ltd.

Contents

Detailed contents

Section 3: Clinical pharmacology   **113**

Section 4: Clinical development   199

Section 5: Statistics and data management   251

Section 8: Therapeutics   417

Preface

This handbook provides a broad overview of all topics relevant to the discipline of pharmaceutical medicine in an accessible and user-friendly format. The breadth of the pharmaceutical medicine curriculum looks daunting, but this book is designed to navigate a path through the mine-field. It will help you with both examinations and gaining a taster of areas of pharmaceutical medicine that are not directly relevant to your current role. Written in the style of the other Oxford Handbook series, it gives the key facts in a concise and readable format, without page upon page of dense text. It is suitable as a revision aid and for quick reference for those working in the pharmaceutical industry or allied fields, those in formal training in pharmaceutical medicine, and other professionals involved in regulatory affairs, clinical research, or the marketing of medicines.

AK
DO'C
PA
January 2013

Contributors

Robert Hemmings
Statistical Assessor,
MHRA, London, UK

Ian Hudson
Director, Licensing Division
MHRA, London, UK

Abigail E Moran
Deputy Manager and
Senior Pharmaceutical Assessor,
MHRA, London, UK

Ruben Pita
Scientific Administrator—Quality
of Medicines,
European Medicines Agency,
London, UK

Rafe Suvarna
Unit Manager, Vigilance and Risk
Management of Medicines Division
(VRMM), MHRA, London, UK

Denise Till
Statistical Assessor,
MHRA, London, UK

John Warren
Director
Medicines Assessment Ltd,
London, UK

Kent Woods
Chief Executive, MHRA,
London, UK

Enver Yousuf
Principal Clinical Advisor, Medsafe
New Zealand Medicines and
Medical Devices Safety Authority,
Wellington, New Zealand

Abbreviations

ABPI	Association of the British Pharmaceutical Industry
ACE	angiotensin-converting-enzyme
ADR	adverse drug reaction
ADME	absorption, distribution, metabolism, and excretion
AE	adverse event
AIMS	Access, Innovation, Mobilization, and Security
ALT	Alanine aminotransferase
ANDA	abbreviated new drug application (US)
ARBS	angiotensin II receptor blockers
ARTG	Australian Register of Therapeutic Goods
AST	Asparate aminotransferase
ATC	anatomical, therapeutic, and chemical classification
ATMP	advanced-therapy medicinal products
AUC	area under the concentration time curve
AZT	Azidothymidine
BLA	biologics license application
BMG	*Bundesministerium für Gesundheit*, Federal Ministry of Health (Germany)
BNF	British National Formulary
BP	British Pharmacopeia
BPH	benign prostatic hypertrophy
BRIC	Brazil, Russia, India, and China
CA	competent authority
CAP	centrally authorized products
CAT	Committee for Advanced Therapies
CBA	cost–benefit analysis
CBER	Center for Biologics Evaluation and Research (US)
CCN	Code Compliance Network
CDE	Centre for Drug Evaluation (China)
CDER	Center for Drug Evaluation and Research (US)
CE	European Conformity
CEN	European Committee for Standardization
CFR	Code of Federal Regulations
CHM	Commission on Human Medicines (UK)
CHMP	Committee for Medicinal Products for Human Use
CI	confidence interval
CIOMS	Council for International Organizations of Medical Sciences

CKD	chronic kidney disease
CL	clearance
Cmax	maximum plasma concentration/peak concentration
CMC	chemistry manufacturing and controls
CMD(h)	Co-ordination Group for Mutual Recognition and Decentralized Procedures (human)
CMS	concerned member state
CNV	copy number variation
COMP	Committee for Orphan Medicinal Products
CONSORT	Consolidated Standards of Reporting Trials
CP	centralized procedure
CPG	clinical practice guidelines
CPMP	Committee for Proprietary Medicinal Products
CPP	certificate of pharmaceutical product
CRA	Clinical Research Associate
CRF	case report form
CRO	clinical research organizations
CSM	Committee on Safety of Medicines
CTA	clinical trial application
CTAg	clinical trial agreements
CTD	common technical document
CTN	clinical trial notification
CTP	clinical trial permission
CUA	cost–utility analysis
CV	curriculum vitae
DCP	decentralized procedure
DDPS	detailed description of pharmacovigilance system
DHPL	Dear Healthcare Professional letter
DIN	drug identification number
DMF	drug master file
DMP	disease management programmes
DMRC	Defective Medicines Report Centre
DPPIV	dipeptidyl peptidase IV
DSMB	Data Safety Monitoring Board
DSRU	Drug Safety Research Unit
DSUR	development safety update report
DUS	drug utilization studies
EAG	Expert Advisory Group
EC	European Commission
ECG	electrocardiogram

ED	effective dose
EDC	electronic data capture
EDQM	European Directorate for the Quality of Medicines & HealthCare
EEA	European Economic Area
EFPIA	European Federation of Pharmaceutical Industries Associations
EFT	embryo-fetal toxicity
EFTA	European Free Trade Association
E&LD	Evaluation and Licensing Division
EMA	European Medicines Agency
ENCePP	The European Network of Centres for Pharmacoepidemiology and Pharmacovigilance
ERA	environmental risk assessment
EPAR	European Public Assessment Report
EPC	European Patent Convention
EPO	European Patent Office
ERB	Ethical Review Board
EthC	Ethics Committee (EU)
EU	European Union
EudraCT	European Union drug regulating authorities Clinical Trials: European clinical trials database
EudraV	Eudra vigilance
FCPA	Foreign Corrupt Practices Act
FDA	Food and Drug Administration (US)
FEED	fertility/early embryonic development
GBA	*Gemeinsamer Bundesausschuss*, Federal Joint Committee (Germany)
GCP	good clinical practice
GDP	good distribution practice
GFR	glomerular filtration rate
GI	gastrointestinal
GLP	good laboratory practice
GLP-1	glucagon-like peptide
GCLP	good clinical laboratory practice
GMP	good manufacturing practice
GMPLA	Good Manufacturing Practice Licensing Authority
GSL	general sales list
GVP	good pharmacovigilance practices
GWAS	genome-wide association studies
HMA	Heads of Medicines Agencies

HMPC	Committee on Herbal Medicinal Products
HPFB	Health Products and Food Branch (of Health Canada)
HRQL	health-related quality of life
HTA	health technology assessment
IB	investigator's brochure
ICH	International Conference on Harmonisation
ICSR	Individual Case Safety Report
IDL	import drug licence
IDMC	Independent Data Monitoring Committee
IEC	Independent Ethics Committee
IFPMA	International Federation of Pharmaceutical Manufacturers and Associations
IFU	Instructions for use
IMP	investigational medicinal product
IND	investigational new drug
INN	international non-proprietary name
INR	international normalized ratio
IP	intellectual property
IQWiG	Institute for Quality and Efficiency in Health Care
IRAS	Integrated Research Application System
IRB	Institutional Review Board
IV	intravenous
IVRS	interactive voice recognition system
JNDA	Japan new drug application
JPMA	Japan Pharmaceutical Manufacturers
KLH	keyhole limpet haemocyanin
KOL	key opinion leader
KW	Kruskal–Wallis test
LML	local manufacturing licence
LOAEL	lowest observed adverse effect level
LREC	Local Research Ethics Committee
MA	marketing authorization
MAA	marketing authorization application
MACE	major adverse cardiovascular endpoints
MAD	mutual acceptance of data
MAH	marketing authorization holder
MaPP	Manual of Policies and Procedures
MCA	Medicines Control Agency (UK)
MDA	Medical Devices Agency (UK)
MDD	Medical Devices Directive

MedDRA	Medical Dictionary for Regulatory Activities
MHLW	Ministry of Health, Labour and Welfare (Japan)
MHRA	Medicines and Healthcare products Regulatory Agency (UK)
MODY	maturity-onset diabetes of the young
MREC	Multi-centre Research Ethics Committee
MRP	mutual recognition procedure
MS	member state
NAS	new active substance
NCA	national competent authorities
NCE	new chemical entity
NDA	new drug application
NICE	National Institute for Health and Clinical Excellence (UK)
NICPBP	National Institute for the Control of Pharmaceutical and Biological Products
NK	natural killer
NNT	number needed to treat
NOAEL	no observed adverse effect level
NOC	notice of compliance
NOCc	NOC granted with conditions
NON	notice of non-compliance
NPV	net present value
NSAID	non-steroidal anti-inflammatory drugs
NYHA	New York Heart Association
OAT	organic anion transporters
OECD	Organization for Economic Co-operation and Development
OMCL	Official Medicines Control Laboratories
OOPD	Office of Orphan Products Development
OTC	over-the-counter products
P	pharmacy medicines
PAES	Post Authorization Safety Study
PAMPA	parallel artificial membrane permeability
PASS	post-authorization safety studies
PD	pharmacodynamics
PDCO	Paediatric Committee
PDUFA	Prescription Drug User Fee Act
PE	pharmacoepidemiology
PFSB	Pharmaceutical and Food Safety Bureau (Japan)
PEM	prescription event monitoring
Ph. Eur.	European Pharmacopoeia

PHRMA	Pharmaceutical Research and Manufacturers of America
PIL	patient information leaflet
PIP	paediatric investigation plans
PL	package leaflet
PK	pharmacokinetic
PMA	Pharmaceutical Manufacturer's Association
PMCPA	Prescription Medicines Code of Practice Authority
PMDA	Pharmaceutical and Medical Devices Agency
POM	prescription-only medicine
PPI	proton pump inhibitor
PPIP	Patient and Public Involvement Programme
PPN	pre- and postnatal development
PRAC	Pharmacovigilance Risk Assessment Committee
PMS	Postmarketing surveillance
PRO	patient reported outcome
PSUR	Periodic Safety Update Report
PT	Prothrombin time
PV	pharmacovigilance
QA	quality assurance
QALY	quality-adjusted life years
QC	quality control
QOL	quality of life
QP	qualified person
QPPV	qualified person responsible for pharmacovigilance
QRD	quality review of document
R&D	research and development
REC	Research Ethics Committee
RCT	randomized control trial
REMS	Risk Evaluation & Mitigation Strategies
RMP	risk management plan
RMS	reference member state
SA	service agreements
SAE	serious adverse event
SAG	Scientific Advisory Group
SAWP	Scientific Advice Working Party
SBD	summary basis of decision
SFDA	State Food and Drug Administration (China)
SIGN	Scottish Intercollegiate Guidelines Network
SmPC	summary of product characteristics
SNDA	supplemental new drug application

SNDS	supplemental new drug submission
SNP	single nucleotide polymorphisms
SOP	standard operating procedures
SPA	special protocol assessment
SmPC	summary of product characteristics
SRBC	sheep red blood cells
SSRI	selective serotonin re-uptake inhibitor
STS	standard toxicity study
SUSAE	suspected unexpected serious adverse event
TD	toxic dose
TDAR	T-cell dependent antibody response
TDM	therapeutic drug monitoring
TGA	Therapeutic Goods Administration (Australia)
TGO	therapeutic goods order
THMP	traditional herbal medicinal (Australia) products
TPP	target product profile
TRIPS	trade-related aspects of intellectual property rights
UKECA	United Kingdom Ethics Committee Authority
Vd	volume of distribution
WHO	World Health Organization
WOCBP	women of child-bearing potential
WMW	Whitney–Mann–Wilcoxon
WTO	World Trade Organization

Section 1

Discovery of new medicines

Chapter 1.1

Intellectual property in discovery

Intellectual property

Intellectual property (IP) refers to various legitimate methods of protecting a product against competition. Common types of IP include:
- Design rights (protect the look of 3D shapes).
- Trademarks (protect logos that distinguish goods).
- Copyrights (protect material that is written down or recorded).
- Patents (protect processes).

Patent

A patent is a legal title that protects an invention from legitimate competition for a limited period of time in a defined geographical territory. To be patentable, an invention must be novel, industrially applicable, and involve an inventive step. An invention may be a process or a product, and an explicit definition of the invention, the so-called 'claims', must be described in any application. Not all things are patentable (e.g. scientific theories and mathematical methods are excluded). To be new, an invention must not have been disclosed publicly before filing. A patent is usually valid for up to 20 years from the date of filing of the application. The granting of a patent helps companies recoup research and development costs, and may be key for raising venture capital. The patent system also promotes knowledge sharing and patents are a good source of technical information (European Patent Office's publication server).

Filing a patent

A patent is granted following an application to a patent office. A patent should be filed at the earliest opportunity, and it is critical that details of the invention are kept secret before the application is filed. The patent application process is structured, and certain procedural steps must be completed within specific time frames. Fees are normally payable. Applications may be made separately in one country, more than one country, or submitted under an international convention (e.g. European Patent Convention). The submitted application is examined by the appropriate patent office and a typical application will consist of:
- A title and abstract.
- A detailed description of the invention indicating how it is used, explicit definitions, drawings, and other relevant technical data.
- What the potential benefits are compared with what is already known or exists, with examples to support the claims in practice.
- The overall scope and justification of the claims. The claims are judged according to the knowledge in the public domain before the date of filing.

European patent process

In the European Union (EU), patent protection is provided by national patents granted by member states or by patents granted by the European Patent Office (EPO) under the European Patent Convention (EPC). An Application under the EPC currently results in separate national patents in each of the designated states. There is no single patent for all European community countries. However, there are proposals for the creation of a so called 'unitary community patent'. The European Patent Organization is an intergovernmental organization set up in 1977 under the EPC. The organization currently has 38 member states, which includes all members of the EU. The European Patent Organization consists of two bodies:

- Administrative Council, which acts in a supervisory role and is composed of representatives of the organization member states.
- EPO, which is supervised by the Administrative Council and provides a uniform patent application procedure.

European Patent Office

The EPO conducts its business in one of the three official languages (English, French, or German). From filing, the procedure lasts on average 3–5 years. An application will be assigned to a Patent Office Examiner who is familiar with the technology described. The Application process comprises:

- Formalities examination.
- Search report (search of databases to ensure that the claims are novel and inventive, whether anything was publically known before the date of filing).
- Substantive examination (the claims and the breadth of the claims are examined to see if the patentability criteria are met).

If the patentability criteria are met, a patent can be granted. If the criteria are not met, the examination report details the concerns and objections to the applicant, who has a period of time to respond. If the examining division is of the opinion that a patent cannot be granted, it will refuse the application. Refused applications can be appealed before the boards of appeal. Following granting of a patent, there follows a 9-month period in which third parties are entitled to file a reasoned notice of opposition. This may result in the patent being maintained as granted, amended, or revoked. The decision taken in the opposition proceedings may also be appealed. Granting of a patent gives rights to prevent others from exploiting the invention and it is the patent holders' responsibility to enforce the patent by challenging violations. Patent holders may, however, choose to license the invention to others in return for financial compensation.

Further reading

꩜ http://www.ipo.gov.uk/
꩜ http://www.epo.org/
꩜ http://ec.europa.eu/internal_market/indprop/patent/index_en.htm

Targeted drug discovery: receptor-based approaches

Agonists/antagonists/enzyme inhibitors

Agonist, antagonist, and enzyme inhibitor approaches are all employed in drug discovery, with genomics, metabolomics, and proteomics helping to deliver potential targets.

The systemic effects of agonists or antagonists may also be further studied with knockout animal approaches. The Cre loxP approach works by introducing loxP sequences of DNA either side of the target gene. Cre-recombinase can then be used to remove the target gene in a knock-out animal, and a similar approach used to introduce extra genes in a knock in animal.

Where hepatic enzyme agonism or antagonism is the goal, sophisticated in vitro systems now exist for testing the effect of drug targets. In vitro models of gut membrane transport have also been developed for absorption studies.

Genomics

Genomics-based approaches to drug discovery centre on evaluating differences in gene expression in the diseased versus the healthy state. These lead to identification of one or usually a number of genes, which when expressed or not expressed lead to changes in the functional status of the individual.

Examples of single gene disorders where specific genes have been identified, and their function characterized include haemochromatosis, Maturity-onset Diabetes of the Young (MODY), and cystic fibrosis. For other disorders, such as Type 2 diabetes, it is likely that a complex interaction across a number of different genes leads to the development of the condition.

Chip based approaches, such as the Affimetrix® chip which measures expression of mRNA, have led to rapid advances in this field.

Proteomics

A limitation of genomics is that measurement of mRNA is inexact as to how much of the mRNA is translated to functional protein production, and what happens to the protein produced to activate it/inactivate it, e.g. glycation or phosphorylation.

For this reason proteomics significantly adds to information about potential drug discovery targets, giving information about expression of different proteins/peptides in the healthy or diseased state, information on their level of function, and whether alterations are seen in post-translational modification.

Computational biology has improved the throughput of targets identified by proteomics into drugs which can be brought into the clinic. A prime example is glivec, a tyrosine kinase inhibitor, which was a first, 'designer' drug, where the enzyme inhibitor was designed to fit the enzyme with the use of 3D modelling techniques.

Metabolomics

Metabolomics are combined with genomics and proteomics to give a snapshot of cellular physiology in the diseased and healthy state. Metabolomics is the measurement of the range of metabolites produced by a given group of cells or tissue. It raises the possibility of targeting enzymes responsible for accumulation of metabolites considered toxic in the diseased state.

Further reading

🔊 www.genomicsdirectory.com
🔊 http://metlin.scripps.edu/
🔊 http://www.genome.gov/10005834

Chapter 1.3

In vitro and in vivo testing of new compounds

Overview

The package of in vitro and in vivo testing required before progression to studies in humans is well described. These include a battery of in vitro tests to assess potential therapeutic effect and toxicity, and in vivo pre-clinical testing to assess therapeutic and reproductive effects.

In vitro testing

- Physiochemical screening; This includes tests of solubility, lipophylicity, and chemical stability.
- Absorption testing: Parallel artificial membrane permeability (PAMPA) assay and Caco-2 (permeability across a single intestinal cell layer), allow for in vitro testing of absorption.
- Distribution testing: Distribution testing focuses on testing of active transport mechanisms, and protein binding. Recommended active transporters which can be screened for interaction in vitro include: P-gp, BCRP, OATP1B1, OATP1B3, OCT2, BSEP, OCT1, OAT1, and OAT3. Plasma protein binding can also be estimated in vitro.
- Hepatocyte screens: Human liver microsomes are used to test for inhibition or activation of the 7 most important CYP450 enzymes (CYP1A, CYP2B6, CYP2C8, CYP2C9, CYP2C19, CYP2D6, and CYP3A4).

Typical tool compounds for P450 testing (see Table 1.3.1)

Genotoxicity screens: Three conventionally used screens exist, the Comet test which utilizes single cell gell electrophoresis, the Ames test which determines if a chemical is a mutagen for salmonella, and the mutatox test which utilizes chemoluminescent *Vibrio* bacteria.

Table 1.3.1 Typical tool compounds for P450 testing

Isoform	Substrate reaction	Positive control inhibitor
CYP1A	Ethoxyresorufin O-deethylation	α-Naphthoflavone
CYP2B6	Bupropion hydroxylation	Ticlopidine
CYP2C8	Paclitaxel 6α-hydroxylation	Montelukast
CYP2C9	Tolbutamide 4-hydroxylation	Sulphaphenazole
CYP2C19	S-mephenytoin 4-hydroxylation	Tranylcypromine
CYP2D6	Dextromethorphan O-demethylation	Quinidine
CYP3A4	Midazolam 1-hydroxylation	Ketoconazole
CYP3A4	Testosterone 6β-hydroxylation	Ketoconazole

Acute toxicity studies in animals

Two species by different routes of administration, one by the IV route to ensure adequate systemic exposure, one by the proposed route of administration. This would also incorporate estimation of the maximum repeatable dose and an assessment of local irritancy.

Repeat dose toxicity in animals

Rodent and non-rodent species required according to guidelines. Duration of test depends on clinical exposure in humans, but at least two 14-day studies are required before progression to man. These studies are carried out via the proposed clinical route.

Reproductive toxicity

Embryo/fetal development carried out in two species, is not required in Europe initially or in Japan if first human studies do not include women of reproductive potential, but this will still need to be conducted at a later date.

Further reading

🔊 http://www.ema.europa.eu/docs/en_GB/document_library/Scientific_guideline/2010/05/WC500090112.pdf

🔊 http://www.emea.europa.eu/docs/en_GB/document_library/Scientific_guideline/2009/09/WC500002720.pdf

Lead optimization

Overview

Lead optimization is the process of drug discovery where the objective is to synthesize new lead compounds which more accurately reflect the desired drug profile. This process is designed to:
- Improve potency.
- Reduce off-target activity.
- Improve physiochemical/metabolic properties, suggesting in vivo pharmacokinetics will be acceptable.

This optimization is accomplished through chemical modification of the of an initial compound structure which is known to have activity at the required target, with modifications chosen by employing structure–activity analysis and structure-based design if structural information about the target is available.

A great deal of information is known about basic changes which can significantly improve characteristics of an agent.
  Examples include:
- Improving half-life: Native GLP-1, which binds to the GLP-1 receptor has a half-life of only a few minutes. Addition of a modification which includes a free-fatty chain leads to association with human albumin and increases half-life by a number of hours.
- Improving enzyme selectivity: DPPIV is an enzyme responsible for the cleavage of GLP-1, contributing to its short half-life. Inhibition of the enzyme can significantly prolong the half-life of GLP-1 but off target inhibition may also occur with respect to DPPII, 8 and 9. This is thought to lead to unpredictable toxicity with respect to autoimmune phenomena.

Experiments for lead optimization
Experiments for lead optimization include in vitro and in vivo pharmacology, stability and solubility assessments, in vitro drug metabolism and delivery, preliminary animal pharmacokinetics, and in vitro and acute toxicology.

Specific steps include:
In vitro pharmacology
- Expansion of drug discovery results.
- Determination of IC50 and IC90 values.

In vivo pharmacology
- Definition and characterization of relevant animal models.
- Determination of ED50 and ED10 values and therapeutic ratio.

Early formulation evaluations
- Analytical chemistry method development and characterization.
- Early formulation definition and assessments.
- Stability and solubility testing versus requirements.

In vitro metabolism
- P-450 Isozymes, microsomes, and/or hepatocytes panel testing.
- Phase II metabolism evaluation.
- Species–species comparisons.

In vitro delivery

Evaluation using in vitro models of:

- GI absorption and example absorption profiles.
- Blood brain barrier passage.
- Skin and other membrane absorption profiles.

Preliminary animal pharmacokinetics:

- Bioanalytical chemistry method development and characterization.
- Preliminary protein binding experiments.
- Pharmacokinetic experiments and example profiles.
- Examination for metabolites in plasma, urine, bile.

Early toxicology via in vitro experiments utilizing:

- Cell-based systems.
- Microarrays.
- Acute or single-dose toxicology.
- Safety pharmacology.
- Genotoxicity panels.

Chapter 1.5

Natural products and herbal medicines

Natural products

Natural products were, for many years, the only medicines available to man. Modern drug development has its roots in empirical observations made over centuries, where natural remedies with medicinal properties were used to treat human disease (e.g. digoxin from the foxglove plant). Natural products include compounds derived from animals, plants, and microbes.

Natural products or their analogues have been an important source of lead compounds in drug development. Natural product-based drugs cover a wide range of therapeutic areas such as anti-infectives, lipid control agents, immunosuppressants, and anti-cancer agents. These products show a great diversity of chemical structure, with approximately half in keeping with Lipinski's rule of five. Lipinski's rule of five describes the properties and structural features that make molecules more or less 'drug-like' (molecular mass less than 500 Daltons, a maximum of 5 hydrogen bond donors and 10 hydrogen bond acceptors, and a log P of less than 5).

Natural product drug discovery programmes are resource intensive and based on:
- Extraction-library screening.
- Bioassay guided isolation.
- Identification and structure elucidation.
- Large-scale manufacture.

Although natural products have been the foundation for many lead compounds in drug development, research aimed at exploiting natural products for drug discovery has declined over the last two decades. This decline is due to the development and implementation in drug discovery programmes of new technologies, such as combinational chemistry and high throughput screening, where 'hit' identification is more rapid and generally less resource intensive. Another potential issue has been the complex intellectual property rights that may surround natural products, following the agreements reached at the Rio Convention on Biological Diversity (1993), where one of the founding principles is 'fair and equitable sharing of benefits arising from genetic resources'. However, despite the decline, the rich chemical diversity of the natural world continues to be of relevance to modern drug discovery, particularly as only a relatively small proportion of the world's biodiversity has been screened for bioactivity.

Currently, renewed interest in natural products is being driven, in part, by the urgent need for new drugs (e.g. to fight multidrug resistance) and by our growing understanding of the molecular sciences. New approaches to evaluate natural products are becoming established, and include:
- Integration of in silico screening (computer technology use to support lead discovery).
- Breakthroughs in fractionation and structure-determination technologies.
- New methods of activity profiling.
- Exploring leads from traditional medicines.

Herbal medicines

According to the Traditional Herbal Medicinal Products (THMP) Directive 2004/24/EC, a herbal medicinal product is:

> Any medicinal product, exclusively containing as active ingredients one or more herbal substances or one or more herbal preparations, or one or more such herbal substances in combination with one or more such herbal preparations.

The THMP Directive establishes a simplified regulatory approval process for herbal medicines in the EU and a Committee for Herbal Medicinal Products (HMPC) within the European Medicines Agency (EMA). The HMPC's activities include assisting the harmonization of herbal registration procedures and integrating herbal medicinal products into the European regulatory framework.

The EU regulatory framework for market access for herbal products allows for a full marketing authorization, based on the quality, safety, and efficacy of the product (either well-established use or full dossier submission, Directive 2001/83/EC) or a traditional herbal registration, based on the safety (if requested by the competent authority), quality and evidence of sufficiently long traditional use of the product (simplified registration procedure, Directive 2004/24/EC). The simplified registration procedure is a national procedure, carried out by competent authorities of individual member states. The necessary physicochemical, biological and microbiological tests are required and products should comply with quality standards in relevant European/member state Pharmacopoeia monographs.

Further reading

🕮 http://ec.europa.eu/health/human-use/herbal-medicines/index_en.htm

Section 2

Medicines regulation

General principles of medicines regulation

Overview

Medicinal products are heavily regulated in order to protect and promote public health. Government agencies throughout the world have responsibility for supervising medicinal products on their market and regulating the activities of the pharmaceutical industry. In the EU, member states (MS) have one or more competent authorities that have these responsibilities. In addition, the European Medicines Agency (EMA) has responsibility for some products and also co-ordinates activities across Ms. The individual MS authorities and the EMA work together in a regulatory network. In the UK, the competent authority is the Medicines and Healthcare products Regulatory Agency.

Within Europe much of the legislative basis for regulation is at a European level with European Directives transposed into national law, European regulations directly applicable in each EU MS, and, in addition, national legislation, such as the Human Medicines Regulations 2012, in the UK. The European network has also produced extensive guidance to assist applicants.

Drug development is long and complex. Medicines regulation requires approval at a number of stages throughout the development process, and throughout the life of the product on the market. Activities carried out by regulatory agencies include:

- Approval of clinical trials.
- Scientific advice.
- Licences of manufacturers and wholesalers.
- Formal licensing of products.
- Pharmacovigilance in the market place.
- Approving variations and line extensions.
- Inspection of manufacturers, clinical trials, laboratories to ensure standards of good manufacturing practice (GMP), good clinical practice (GCP), good distribution practice (GDP), good laboratory practice (GLP), good pharmacovigilance practices (GVP).
- Monitoring of advertising.
- Taking enforcement action.
- Testing of medicines on the market and surveillance for counterfeits.

Types of products vary enormously, including the latest gene therapy or biotechnology-derived product, other new active substances, established products with new uses, vaccines, generics, parallel imports, herbals, and homeopathic products.

Within the EU, there are a number of regulatory routes for approval of medicines. The majority of new, innovative products are assessed through the centralized procedure, operated by the EMA and its scientific Committee for Medicinal Products for Human Use (CHMP). Members of this committee act as *Rapporteurs* for specific products and will arrange for the assessment of products, generally at their national agency, then present the conclusions back to the CHMP. The centralized process has a number of regulatory options for approval allowing for different circumstances. These include full approval, conditional approval for products to treat life-threatening or seriously debilitating illnesses, and licensing under exceptional circumstances for medicines to treat rare diseases. Reflecting the increasing emphasis on monitoring medicines in the market place, companies need to get approval for risk management plans at the time of the authorization. These plans describe how any safety issues will be monitored and how gaps in knowledge of the product will be filled. Many approvals are associated with commitments from the company to submit further data to supplement the extent of knowledge available at the time of approval. The alternatives to the centralized procedure are the decentralized and mutual recognition procedures, run by the Heads of Medicines Agencies. With these procedures, one MS takes a lead role in the assessment (reference member state, RMS) and other MS (concerned member state, CMS) reviews the assessment performed by the lead MS. These procedures are used for the majority of established products and generics.

The formal requirements for licensing and, indeed, throughout the lifecycle of the product are that appropriate standards of quality, safety, and efficacy are met. Regulators review data submitted by applicants and from other sources, and ensure themselves that the benefits of the product outweigh the risk. If safety issues emerge, then regulators will wish to see how risks can be minimized, perhaps by appropriate warnings, communications to health professionals, or by restrictions to licences.

Medicines regulation is a rapidly evolving area. Whilst there are increasing efforts to achieve global standardization of requirements through the International Conference on Harmonisation (ICH) process, there has been a constant stream of new legislation and requirements, including, over recent years, the Clinical Trials Directive, new Paediatric, Advanced Therapies, and Pharmacovigilance regulations.

Other changes have been and will continue to be:
• Greater patient involvement in decision taking.
• Greater openness and transparency.
• Greater dialogue between licensing and health technology assessment bodies.
• Consideration of the methodologies available to assess risk benefit and their applicability to medicines regulation.

As medicines regulation has become ever more complex, there are now some moves to try to simplify the regulatory environment through initiatives, such as the Better Regulation of Medicines Initiative in the UK, the variations regulation in Europe, and the recent approach taken to the regulation of clinical trials in the UK with a more proportionate approach. There is a recognition that regulation needs to take a more risk-based approach, and that the regulatory framework needs to adapt and evolve as new technologies are developed. Regulators recognize they have an important role in helping to facilitate safe innovation, and provide advice to those developing new medicines, in order to facilitate advances in public health.

Chapter 2.2

Medicines regulation in the UK

The Thalidomide tragedy

Thalidomide was marketed in the UK in April 1958 and was promoted for use as an anti-emetic in pregnant women. Subsequently, the use of Thalidomide in pregnancy was shown to be associated with congenital malformations of the limbs (phocomelia) and other internal abnormalities. Thalidomide was withdrawn in 1961, and non-clinical studies would confirm Thalidomide to be a potent teratogen. Prior to the Thalidomide tragedy, there was no legal requirement for the independent testing of a marketed drug with respect to quality, safety, and efficacy. The Thalidomide incident caused a public outcry and, as a direct consequence, the UK government set up Medical Advisory Committees, tasked with determining measures for effective drug regulation.

The Medicines Act (1968)

The Medicines Act of 1968 consolidated existing UK legislation and incorporated principles set by other standards of the time:
• The US Federal Pure Food and Drugs Act (1906).
• The US Federal Food, Drug and Cosmetic Act (1938).
• US New Drug Amendment (the Kefauver–Harris Amendment 1962).
• The EU Council Directive 65/65/EEC (1965).

Since joining the European Community (EC), all European pharmaceutical legislation is transposed into UK national law and the Act has been regularly amended to ensure consistency with EC legalisation. Recently, the Medicines Act and approximately 200 Statutory Instruments have been consolidated into the Human Medicines Regulations 2012 (SI 2012/1916).

UK Regulatory Agency

The Medicines Division was set up in 1972 for the day-to-day administration of the Medicines Act. The Medicines Division evolved into the Medicines Control Agency in 1989, and the Medicines and Healthcare products Regulatory Agency (MHRA) was formed in April 2003, joining and replacing the Medical Devices Agency (MDA) and the Medicines Control Agency (MCA).
• MHRA is an executive agency of the UK Department of Health.
• The Agency's mission statement is to enhance and safeguard the public's health by ensuring that medicines and medical devices meet the highest standards of safety, quality, performance, and effectiveness.
• The Agency is structured into 10 divisions, including licensing division (responsible for assessing and approving marketing authorization applications), vigilance and risk management of medicines (safe use of marketed medicines), and inspection, enforcement and standards (ensuring compliance with standards that apply to the manufacture and supply of medicines).

- A number of independent advisory committees support the work of the MHRA and advise UK Ministers on matters relating to the regulation of medicines and medical devices.

Commission on Human Medicines and expert advisory groups

In 2005, the Commission on Human Medicines (CHM) was formed from the amalgamated responsibilities of the Medicines Commission and the Committee on Safety of Medicines (CSM). The appointment of the Chairman and members (including two lay representatives) are carried out by the NHS Appointments Commission. CHM is supported by a number of expert advisory groups (EAG) covering various therapeutic areas. The duties of the Commission are set out the Human Medicines Regulations and include:

- Advising ministers on matters relating to human medicinal products.
- Advising the licensing authority where the licensing authority has a duty to consult the Commission or where the licensing authority chooses to consult the Commission, including giving advice in relation to the quality, safety, and efficacy of human medicinal products.
- Considering representations made in relation to the Commission's advice (either in writing or at a hearing) by an applicant, or by a licence or marketing authorization holder.
- Promoting the collection and investigation of information relating to adverse reactions for human medicines.

Marketing authorization applications (MAAs)

According to pharmaceutical legislation, a medicinal product may only be placed on the market when the competent authority of a member state for its own territory (national authorization) has issued a marketing authorization or when the EC has granted authorization for the entire community (community authorization).

There are a number of different types of application, and the application type depends on the country the product is going to be marketed in and the type of medicine. MAAs include a national procedure, the mutual recognition procedure (MRP), the decentralized procedure (DCP), and the centralized procedure (CP). Regardless of the procedural type, all applications must be submitted in the common technical document (CTD) format (ICH M4).

Further reading

🔊 http://www.legislation.gov.uk/uksi/2012/1916/made
🔊 www.mhra.gov.uk

Medicines regulation in the EU

Pharmaceutical legislation

In 1952, six countries signed the Treaty of Paris, forming the European Coal and Steel Community. Since then, a number of treaties have been ratified and the EU has evolved, gaining new responsibilities and MSs. According to Article 288 of the Treaty on the Functioning of the EU, to exercise the EU's competences, institutions adopt Regulations, Directives, decisions, recommendations, and opinions (see Table 2.3.1 for a list of important pharmaceutical legislation).

• A Regulation has general applications, is binding in its entirety, and is directly applicable in all MSs.
• A Directive is binding as to the result to be achieved, but leaves to the national authorities the choice of form and methods of implementation. Directives must be transposed into national law.

Pharmaceutical legislation has significantly evolved since the first European pharmaceutical Directive was adopted in 1965 (Directive 65/65/EEC), and medicines regulation is now consolidated in Directive 2001/83/EC (as amended). The legislation on medicinal products is applicable to the European Economic Area (EEA) States: 27 member states of the EU plus Iceland, Liechtenstein, and Norway.

Medicinal products

Medicinal products for human use may only be placed on the market in the EU if a marketing authorization has been issued by the EC or by a competent authority of an MS. In Directive 2001/83/EC, a medicinal product is defined as:

• Any substance or combination of substances presented as having properties for treating or preventing disease in human beings; or
• Any substance or combination of substances which may be used in or administered to human beings either with a view to restoring, correcting or modifying physiological functions by exerting a pharmacological, immunological or metabolic action, or to making a medical diagnosis.

Marketing authorization procedures in the EU

Marketing authorizations can be obtained by four procedural routes, three National authorization procedures (established in Directive 2001/83/EC) and one Union authorization procedure (established in Regulation (EC) 726/2004) (see Table 2.3.2 for more details on these procedures):

• National Application: a marketing authorization application (MAA) is submitted by an applicant in one MS.
• Mutual Recognition Procedure (MRP): a marketing authorization (MA) exists in an MS (the country is called the reference member state [RMS] during the procedure). An MAA is submitted in a number of

MS (concerned member states [CMS]) and following assessment, CMS agree to 'recognize' the MA in the RMS within 90 days (unless a 'risk to public health' is raised). Divergent opinions are resolved by referral.

- Decentralized procedure (DCP): no previous national MA has been granted in any MS, and the applicant submits an MAA simultaneously in a selected RMS and CMS. The RMS takes the lead in the assessment of the dossier for this 210-day procedure and divergent opinions are resolved by referral.

A referral is the formal mechanism used to resolve divergent opinions between MS and the Heads of Agencies Coordination Group for Mutual Recognition and Decentralized Procedures (human) [CMD(h)]—facilitates resolution of conflicting views.

- Centralized procedure (CP) was established under Regulation (EC) 726/2004 and it is a mandatory procedure for medicinal products in the following areas: biotechnology, HIV/AIDS, oncology, diabetes, neurodegenerative disorders, autoimmune diseases and other immune dysfunctions, viral diseases, officially designated 'orphan medicinal products', and may be used for 'others' deemed of significant therapeutic, scientific, or technical innovation, or if the authorization would be in the interest of public health and generics of centrally authorized medicinal products.
- The initial assessment of the MAA is carried out by two MS designated as *Rapporteur* and *Co-Rapporteur*. These MS are selected on the basis of their expertise by the EMA, not by the applicant. The assessment process follows a 210 day timetable. It is the CHMP, a scientific committee of the EMA, that is responsible for reaching the final decision on whether the benefit risk balance is positive or negative Approval can be given in full, as a conditional approval or as an approval in exception circumstances. CHMP opinion is then conveyed to the European Commission (EC), which is ultimately responsible for issuing a formal decision on marketing of the product. Once granted by the EC, a centralized (Community) marketing authorization is valid in all EU states. Following the grant, the EMA publishes a full scientific assessment report called a European Public Assessment Report (EPAR).

Further reading

🔗 http://ec.europa.eu/health/documents/eudralex/index_en.htm
🔗 http://www.hma.eu

Table 2.3.1 Important pharmaceutical legislation

Directives and Regulations	Topic
Directive 65/65/EC	Medicines
Directive 2001/83/EC	Medicines
Directive 2003/63/EC	Medicines
Regulation 726/2004	Medicines
Directive 2011/62/EU	Falsified medicinal products
Directive 2001/20/EC	Clinical trials
Directive 2005/28/EC	GCP
Regulation 1235/2010	Pharmacovigilance
Directive 2010/84/EU	Pharmacovigilance
Regulation 1234/2008	Variations
Directive 92/28/EC	Advertising
Regulation 141/2000	Orphan medicinal products
Regulation 1901/2006	Paediatrics
Regulation 1902/2006	Paediatrics
Regulation 1394/2007	Advanced therapies
Directive 93/42/EC	Medical devices
Directive 90/385/EC	Active implantable devices
Directive 98/79/EC	In vitro diagnostics
EU Legislation–Eudralex	
Volume 1	Pharmaceutical legislation of medicinal products for human use
Volume 2	Pharmaceutical legislation Notice to Applicants and regulatory guidelines medicinal products for human use
Volume 3	Scientific guidelines for medicinal products for human use
Volume 4	GMP guidelines
Volume 5	Pharmaceutical legislation of medicinal products for veterinary use
Volume 6	Notice to Applicants and regulatory guidelines for medicinal products for veterinary use
Volume 7	Scientific guidelines for medicinal products for veterinary use
Volume 8	Maximum residue limits guidelines (MRL)
Volume 9	Pharmacovigilance guidelines
Volume 10	Clinical trials guidelines

Table 2.3.2 Marketing authorization procedures in the EU

Mutual recognition procedure (MRP)		Decentralized procedure (DCP)		Centralized procedure (CP)	
Day 0	Reference member state (RMS) circulates assessment report (AR) to concerned member states (CMSs)	Day 0	Part I—procedure starts	Day 0	Procedure starts
Day 50	AR reviewed by CMSs and comments and position communicated to RMS/CMS and applicant	Day 70	RMS circulates a Day 70 AR to CMSs and applicant	Day 80	Assessment Reports from the Rapporteur and the Co-Rapporteur circulated to CHMP members and applicant
Day 60	Response to comments provided by the applicant	Day 100	CMS circulated comments to RMS/CMS and applicant	Day 100	Comments from peer reviewers and CHMP members
Day 60–85	Resolution of outstanding issues—break-out meeting	Day 105	Day 105 Clock-stop letter	Day 120	Overall conclusions and List of Questions adopted by CHMP AR sent to the applicant
Day 85	CMS inform RMS and applicant of any outstanding issues and position		Clock-off period—applicant prepares responses to List of Questions		Clock-off period—applicant prepares responses to List of Questions
Day 90	End of procedure—Mutual Recognition or If consensus not reached between member states—referral to CMD(h)	Day 106	Part II—valid submission of Responses Clock re-start	Day 121	Valid submission of Responses Clock re-start
		Day 120	RMS circulates a Day 120 AR, following assessment of the applicant's responses	Day 150	Rapporteur/Co-Rapporteur joint assessment of responses circulated to CHMP members and applicant

(Continued)

Table 2.3.2 (Continued)

Mutual recognition procedure (MRP)	Decentralized procedure (DCP)		Centralized procedure (CP)	
	Day 145	CMS circulated comments to RMS/CMS and applicant	Day 170	Comments from CHMP members
	Day 150	If consensus reached, RMS closes procedure	Day 180	CHMP discussion and decision on need to adopt a List of Outstanding Issues and/or Oral Explanation by applicant
		If consensus not reached, outstanding points sent to applicant		Clock-off period—if necessary
	By Day 160	Applicant submits responses	Day 210	CHMP opinion and CHMP AR adopted—opinion communicated to EC for ratification
	By Day 180	RMS updates AR		
	Up to Day 195	Breakout meeting (CMD(h) informed)		
	Day 210	Consensus: Approval or Non-Approval		
		No consensus—divergent opinions: referral to CMD(h)		

The European Medicines Agency and Heads of Medicines Agencies

The European Medicines Agency (EMA)

The EMA (formerly the European Medicines Evaluation Agency [EMEA]) was established in Canary Wharf, London in 1995 in accordance with Council Regulation (EEC) No 2309/93. The EMA is a decentralized agency of the European Union and the Agency aims to foster scientific excellence in the evaluation and supervision of medicines, for the benefit of public and animal health. The Agency co-ordinates the scientific resources put at its disposal by competent authorities (a network of over 4500 national experts). These experts are members of the Agency's scientific committees and assessment teams and the Agency is responsible for the scientific evaluation of marketing authorization applications submitted via the CP.

Scientific evaluation is performed by a number of Committees with different roles and each committee is composed of members from EU and EEA states:

- Committee for Medicinal Products for Human Use (CHMP): this replaced the former Committee for Proprietary Medicinal Products (CPMP). It is responsible for preparing the Agency's opinions on all questions concerning medicines for human use in accordance with Regulation (EC) No 726/2004. The CHMP consults and is supported by its Working Parties and Scientific Advisory Groups (SAG). CHMP plays an important role in:
  - EU-wide pharmacovigilance activities;
  - issuing urgent safety restrictions due to emerging safety concerns;
  - Assessment of Marketing Authorization Applications submitted via the CP and publishing an EPAR;
  - in arbitration procedures following unresolved referrals in MRP and DCP;
  - provision of protocol assistance/scientific advice;
  - preparation of scientific and regulatory guidelines for the pharmaceuticals industry.
- Committee for Orphan Medicinal Products (COMP): responsible for reviewing applications from sponsors seeking 'orphan medicinal product designation' and for advising the EC on matters relating to orphan products.
- Committee on Herbal Medicinal Products (HMPC): replaced the CPMP Working Party on Herbal Medicinal Products. HMPC assists in the harmonization of procedures and provisions concerning herbal medicines.
- Paediatric Committee (PDCO): assess the content of paediatric investigation plans (PIP) and adopts opinions.
- Committee for Advanced Therapies (CAT): assesses the quality, safety, and efficacy of advanced-therapy medicinal products (ATMPs), preparing draft opinions on ATMP applications.
- Pharmacovigilance Risk Assessment Committee (PRAC): responsible for all aspects of risk management of medicines.

Heads of Medicines Agencies

The Heads of Medicines Agencies (HMA) is a network of the Heads of the National competent authorities. Competent authorities are organizations who are responsible for the regulation of medicinal products for human use in the European Economic Area. The HMA is supported by working groups and by the HMA Management Group and Permanent Secretariat. The HMA co-operates with the EMA and the EC in the operation of the European Medicines Regulatory Network.

The HMA works to foster an effective and efficient European Medicines Regulatory System and aims to protect and promote public and animal health in Europe. The HMA has the responsibility for the MRP and DCP, and focuses on the development, co-ordination, and consistency of the European Medicines Regulatory System. The HMA CMDh has the following responsibilities:

- Divergent opinions between the MS involved in a MRP or DCP are considered by CMDh. CMDh attempts to reach consensus within a 60-day assessment procedure.
- CMDh aims to ensure consistency of standards and good quality decision making across the EU in the interests of public health.
- CMDh aims to achieve the harmonization of summary of product characteristics of nationally authorized products in cases that would benefit citizens of the Community.
- CMDh aims to present a harmonized view on the interpretation of Directives and Regulations.

Further reading

ℛ http://www.ema.europa.eu/
ℛ http://www.hma.eu/

The European Directorate for the Quality of Medicines and HealthCare, European Pharmacopoeia, and British Pharmacopoeia

The European Directorate for the Quality of Medicines and HealthCare

The European Directorate for the Quality of Medicines and HealthCare (EDQM) is a Directorate of the Council of Europe, located in Strasbourg, France. The EDQM is involved in the harmonization and co-ordination of standardization, regulation, and quality control of medicines, blood transfusion, organ transplantation, pharmaceuticals, and pharmaceutical care. The EDQM is structured into a number of divisions and departments, and has responsibilities that include:

- The promotion and protection of human and animal health.
- Preparation, establishment, and distribution of chemical and biological reference standards.
- Co-ordination of the European network of Official Medicines Control Laboratories (OMCL).
- Co-ordination of activities for the elaboration of guidelines and recommendations for organ transplantation and blood transfusion.
- Co-ordination of activities for ensuring the quality of medicines.
- The technical secretariat of the European Pharmacopoeia Commission.
- Evaluation of applications for Certificates of Suitability of the Monographs of the European Pharmacopoeia.
- Publication and distribution of the European Pharmacopoeia.

The European Pharmacopoeia

The European Pharmacopoeia (Ph. Eur.) is a reference work for the quality control of medicines in Europe. It is maintained and published by the EDQM. The official standards published by the Ph. Eur. provide a legal and scientific framework for the quality control of medicines. The Ph. Eur. contains monographs for a wide range of active substances, excipients, and general test methods. These specifications concern qualitative and quantitative composition, the raw materials used in production, and the intermediates of synthesis. All producers of medicines or substances for pharmaceutical use must apply the standards of the Ph. Eur. and demonstrating compliance with these standards is a necessary aspect of a marketing authorization application for a medicinal product. The European Pharmacopoeia can be used by manufacturers and National and European health authorities to check the quality of medicines. Biological products and vaccines, blood and plasma derivatives and radiopharmaceutical preparations are also covered by the Ph. Eur.

The European Pharmacopoeia aims are:

- Ensure the same quality of medicines for all EU citizens.
- Provision of recognized quality standards for medicinal substances.
- Facilitate free movement, trade and access of medicines.
- Respond quickly to new potential risks to public health.

The British Pharmacopeia

The British Pharmacopoeia (BP) is updated annually by the British Pharmacopoeia Commission Secretariat (part of the MHRA). The BP is the official collection of standards for UK medicinal products and pharmaceutical substances. The monographs of the Ph. Eur. are reproduced in the BP. The volumes of the BP contain general notices, test methods, and monographs that set out the standards for:

- Medicinal substances.
- Excipients.
- Widely used unlicenced medicines.
- Formulated preparations.
- Blood-related products.
- Immunological products.
- Radiopharmaceutical preparations.
- Surgical materials.
- Homeopathic preparations.
- Infrared reference spectra.

Further reading

෴ http://www.edqm.eu/site/Homepage-628.html
෴ http://www.pharmacopoeia.co.uk/

The Food and Drug Administration

The Food and Drug Administration

The Food and Drug Administration (FDA) is an Agency within the US Department of Health and Human Services, responsible for protecting and advancing public health. In relation to medicines, the Office of Medical Products and Tobacco provides co-ordination for the centres of drugs, biologics and medical devices:
- Center for Drug Evaluation and Research (CDER).
- Center for Biologics Evaluation and Research (CBER).
- Office of Special Medical Programs.
- Center for Devices and Radiological Health.
- Office of Combination Products.
- Office of Good Clinical Practice.
- Office of Orphan Product Development.
- Office of Paediatric Therapeutics.

Advisory committees

The FDA utilizes 50 committees and panels to obtain independent expert advice on scientific, technical, and policy matters. Advisory committees may recommend approval or non-approval of a marketing application. The FDA generally follows an advisory committee's recommendation, but is not obliged to do so.

US drug regulation milestones

Medicines Regulation is covered by the Federal Food, Drug and Cosmetic Act, which has undergone numerous amendments since its origins in 1938. Section 21 of the Code of Federal Regulations (CFR) contains most of the regulations pertaining to medicinal products.
- 1938: Food, Drug and Cosmetic Act required drug safety testing before marketing.
- 1962: Kefauver–Harris amendments to the Food, Drug and Cosmetic Act set the standard for modern drug regulation: 'Drugs were to be safe and effective, based on substantial evidence, consisting of adequate and well-controlled trials, conducted by experts qualified by scientific training and experience'.
- 1982: Waxman–Hatch Act (Drug Price Competition and Patent Term Restoration Act) allows applications for marketing generic versions of brand-name drugs without conducting duplicative clinical studies.
- 1983: Orphan Drug Act.
- 1992: Prescription Drug User Fee Act (PDUFA) authorizes the FDA to collect fees from companies.
- 1997: Food and Drug Administration Modernization Act (FDAMA).
- 2002: Best Pharmaceuticals for Children Act.
- 2007: the Food and Drug Administration Amendments Act.

Types of applications

Investigational new drug (IND) application

There are three types of IND and two IND categories (commercial and non-commercial). The IND application must contain information on animal pharmacology and toxicology studies, manufacturing information, and clinical protocols and investigator information:

- Investigator IND is submitted by a physician who both initiates and conducts an investigation.
- Emergency use IND allows the FDA to authorize the use of an experimental drug in an emergency.
- Treatment IND is for an experimental drug that shows promise in clinical testing for serious or immediately life-threatening conditions.

New drug application (NDA)

The NDA application is the means by which an applicant formally proposes that the FDA approve a new pharmaceutical for sale and marketing in the US. The Manual of Policies and Procedures (MaPPs) is a collection of approved CDER instructions to help standardized the drug review process. The review process will determine whether the manufacturing methods are adequate to preserve the quality of the drug, whether the proposed labelling is appropriate and whether the drug is safe and effective (the benefits outweigh the risks). Three distinct approaches are available for drugs that treat serious diseases; fast track, priority review, and accelerated approval. Changes to a product that have already been approved are requested using a supplemental NDA (SNDA).

Abbreviated new drug application (ANDA)

An ANDA provides the route for review and approval of a generic medicinal product. Applicants must scientifically demonstrate that their product is comparable (bioequivalent) to an innovator product.

Biologics license application (BLA)

Both CDER and CBER have regulatory responsibility for therapeutic biological products. The types of products subject to BLA include monoclonal antibodies, cytokines, growth factors, and enzymes (CDER).

Drug applications for over-the-counter (OTC) drugs

An OTC drug monograph is developed and published in the Federal Register and new products that conform to the monograph may be marketed without the need for FDA pre-approval. However, OTC drugs that do not conform must submit an NDA.

Further reading

ॐ http://www.fda.gov/Drugs

Chapter 2.7

Health Canada

Health Canada

Health Canada is the Federal Department responsible for drug and device regulation in Canada. The Federal Department of Health was established in 1919 and the Food and Drugs Act, the law that governs the drug and food regulatory system was introduced in 1920. There have been a number of amendments/revisions to the Act and Regulations, particularly following the Thalidomide tragedy of the 1960s.

An ongoing project at the Agency is the Blueprint for Renewal (including the Progressive Licensing Project), which aims to modernize Canada's regulatory system for health products and food.

Regulatory procedures

Clinical trial application

A sponsor must submit a clinical trial application (CTA) in order to conduct a clinical trial in Canada. The review process for CTA is carried out by Health Canada's Health Products and Food Branch (HPFB). As with other jurisdictions, clinical trials must be conducted in accordance with GCP and the HPFB has the authority to conduct inspections of clinical trials to ensure compliance.

New drug submission (NDS), abbreviated new drug submission (ANDS), and supplemental new drug submission (SNDS)

For new drug applications, applicants submit either an NDS or an ANDS for generic medicinal products. Certain NDSs may be processed more quickly if they are designated priority review status. Priority review may be granted to a NDS if the product represents a significant benefit over existing therapies or if no product is currently marketed in Canada. If following review a positive risk benefit opinion is reached, a Notice of Compliance (NOC) is issued. Conversely, a Notice of Non-compliance (NON) is issued when the HPFB finds that the risk benefit is negative.

An NOC certifies that a medicinal product complies with the Food and Drugs Act and Regulations and that the risk benefit profile is considered favourable. An NOC may be granted with conditions (NOCc) for drugs treating life-threatening diseases. Conditions are specific follow-up measures. Additional studies usually required to confirm clinical benefit.

Once a company has received an NOC, the drug can be marketed in Canada for a specific use and Health Canada issues a Summary Basis of Decision (SBD). The SBD outlines the factors that lead to the decision to grant a marketing authorization (regulatory, quality, efficacy, and safety information). Changes to already authorized products are made by submitting an SNDS. All marketed drugs must have an eight digit drug identification number (DIN).

Further reading

🔊 http://www.hc-sc.gc.ca/index-eng.php

Chapter 2.8

Medsafe and the Therapeutic Goods Administration

Regulation of medicines in New Zealand

Medsafe

Medsafe is the New Zealand Medicines and Medical Devices Safety Authority. It is part of the Ministry of Health and administers the Medicines Act 1981. Although part of the Ministry, Medsafe receives the majority of funding from fees.

Medicines regulation

The Medicines Act 1981 regulates the manufacture, sale, and supply of medicines in New Zealand. The Act defines a medicine under Section 3. In practical terms, a product is defined as a medicine if it is administered to humans for a therapeutic purpose. Section 4 defines therapeutic purpose and includes the treatment, diagnosis, and prevention of disease or the modification of a physiological function. The Medicines regulations 1984 lay out the data requirements for an application for consent to distribute a medicine. The regulations also define the standards with regard to the product information and labelling.

In order for a medicine to be marketed in New Zealand, an application with supporting documentation must be made for the Minister of Health to give consent. In practice, an application is made to the regulatory authority who advises the Minister (or their delegate) on whether an application should be granted consent.

Regulation of medicines in Australia

Therapeutic Goods Administration (TGA)

The TGA is part of the Australian Government Department of Health and Ageing and administers the Therapeutic Goods Act, together with associated regulations and orders. Any product for which therapeutic claims are made must be listed or registered on the Australian Register of Therapeutic Goods (ARTG) before it may be supplied in Australia.

Medicines regulation

The Therapeutic Goods Act 1989 sets out in law a system of controls relating to the quality, safety, efficacy, and timely availability of therapeutic goods that are used in Australia (including those produced overseas) or are exported from Australia. The Therapeutic Goods Regulations 1990 provide further detail to the Act, specifying the specific requirements necessary to comply with the Act.

Therapeutic goods orders (TGOs)

A number of TGOs supplement the Act and Regulations. The orders set out the standards for items regulated under the Act. For example, TGO 69 sets out the general requirements for labels for medicines. A number of orders exist that revoke or amend older orders.

Towards a joint regulatory scheme

The New Zealand prime minister announced the decision to proceed with the Australia New Zealand Therapeutics Products Agency during an address to the Australian Parliament in July 2011. Establishment of the agency was expected to take at least 5 years, but during this time it is expected that increased collaboration between the two regulators would take place.

Further reading

℞ http://www.medsafe.govt.nz/
℞ http://www.tga.gov.au/industry/pm.htm

Medicines regulation in Japan

Overview

Regulatory responsibilities in Japan are undertaken by a number of regulatory authorities; these include the Ministry of Health Labour and Welfare (MHLW), Pharmaceutical and Food Safety Bureau (PFSB), and the Evaluation and Licensing Division (E&LD), which grants orphan status, priority or accelerated review, and approvals. These interact with a fourth independent agency, the Pharmaceutical and Medical Devices Agency (PMDA), which itself contains an evaluation centre including 7 new drug evaluation divisions and 2 safety divisions.

Pharmaceutical and Medical Devices Agency (PMDA)

The PMDA fulfils a number of roles, both during clinical trials, post Japan new drug application (JNDA) submission, and with respect to monitoring post marketing safety.

PMDA consultations

Not mandatory, but highly recommended in early stages of clinical development, especially when multinational studies are considered. Formal consultation points occur pre-phase I, pre-phase II, pre-late phase II, end of phase II and pre-JNDA. The preliminary and additional consultations are informal, non-minuted, and free. Consultations in writing are possible, as are those to review the whole development strategy and proposed JNDA package in advance. Consultations on multi-national phase III studies are also encouraged.

Timing of PMDA consultations

- Two months between application and meeting.
- Dossier submitted 5 weeks before meeting.
- PMDA opinion issued 4 days prior to the meeting, to which the applicant responds, with unresolved issues discussed at the meeting itself.
- External experts can attend the meeting on behalf of the applicant.

Pilot consultations

Pilot pre-assessment consultations are currently running, evaluating data quality, non-clinical and early phase data prior to formal submission. These are designed to shorten the review process and reduce the workload on the applicant. Another pilot consultation programme is running with respect to biomarkers and pharmacogenomics advice.

Clinical trial notifications

Clinical trial notifications (CTNs) are mandatory for all stages of development. The process for the first is completed within 30 days, subsequent ones finish within 14 days.

Japan new drug application (JNDA)

Review times for the JNDA currently stand at around 15 months for priority review products and around 22 months for standard review. The target by 2012 is to shorten these to 9 and 12 months, respectively.

Priority reviews

Automatically granted to orphan drugs and medical devices. Granted to other drugs and medical devices according to the seriousness of the underlying condition to be treated, and the perceived utility of the intervention.

Orphan drugs

Condition being treated must be serious and rare, with less than 50,000 patients in Japan. There must be no alternative treatment, or it must be significantly safer and more efficacious than existing options. The development plan must be feasible. Priority review, extension of the re-examination period, and reduced PMDA fees, coupled with tax breaks, are all advantages. HIV drugs are considered special orphan drugs, and the US NDA or EU MAA can be submitted.

Re-examination

MHLW designates a re-examination period of 8 years for new chemical entity (NCE), 6 years for new prescription combination drugs, 4 years for new indications or remaining time of original examination period (whichever is longer), and 10 years for orphan drugs. PMS data is used in the re-examination process, and generics applications cannot be submitted until the re-examination period is over.

Vaccines and biologicals

Specific guidelines exist for the submission of vaccines and biologicals, including advice on such issues as adjuvant requirements and chemistry manufacturing and controls (CMC) guidance.

Future direction of the agency

Policy papers published by the PMDA indicate a willingness for closer collaboration with both China and South Korea with respect to clinical development. The PMDA also plans to encourage Japanese participation in multinational clinical trials.

Further reading

🕸 http://www.pmda.go.jp/english/index.html

Medicines regulation in China

Overview

The agency which handles medicines regulation in China is the SFDA. Whilst it is resource constrained, it undertakes data-driven assessment of potential new medicines via the CDE (Centre for Drug Evaluation). Long review times and some unpredictable outcomes have, however, led to proposals for reform over the next 3 years.

Local product testing is by a government lab, the NICPBP is required for registration of medicines, with stricter regulations involving local batch release applying to biologicals.

Data exclusivity

China complies with the TRIPS agreement on intellectual property, regulations therefore allow for 6 years data exclusivity from the date of marketing authorization. This applies to NCEs and biologicals, to imported or locally manufactured products, but enforcement by the authorities is limited.

Monitoring period

If products are locally manufactured, they are subject to additional protection afforded by a 3–5 year monitoring period, during which no generic can be approved, unless the generic has already passed the IND stage. This rule is applicable to both new chemical entities and to biologicals.

Review process

Submissions are required at both the IND (CTP or clinical trial permission) stage, and the NDA (IDL or import drug licence/LML local manufacturing licence) stage. Separate clinical trials are needed for each indication, and a certificate of pharmaceutical product or CPP is also required.

Classes of drugs

Table 2.10.1 shows the six classes of drugs that exist. Table 2.10.2 shows the clinical trial requirements for licensing, and the number of Chinese patients required for licensing.

Reimbursement in China

China operates a reimbursible drug list, divided into list A and list B, list A being 100% reimbursed, list B 50–95% reimbursed. List A drugs are those for chronic diseases such as hypothyroidism or Type 1 diabetes mellitus. There are national and regional lists; no regional variation is allowed in

Table 2.10.1 Classes of drugs

Class 1	Drug not yet approved internationally nor in China
Class 2	Drug with changed administration route and not yet approved in any country
Class 3	Drug approved internationally but not yet approved in China
Class 4	Drug with changed salt form, but no change in mechanism of action and not yet approved in China
Class 5	Drug with changed dosage form, but no change in administration route
Class 6	Drug substance or preparation following national standard (generic)

Table 2.10.2 Patients required in licensing studies

	Class 1	Class 2	Class 3	Class 4	Class 5	Class 6
Phase I	20–30	20–30	PK	PK	PK	-
Phase II	100	100	-	-	-	-
Phase III	300	300	100	100	100	100
Phase IV	2000	2000	-	-	-	-
Bio Equiv	-	-	-	-	18–24	

List A, but up to 15% variation is allowed in list B. Not only is it vitally important to gain registration in China, but also to gain access to the reimbursement list.

China as a market for the future

China is clearly a vitally important future market for all multi-national pharmaceutical companies given its rapid economic growth and market reforms. As such, given the long lead times for regulatory approval in China, appropriate planning with respect to local clinical trials is crucial at an early stage of the development programme.

Further reading
℞ http://eng.sfda.gov.cn/eng/

Chapter 2.11

Medical device regulation

Definition and classification of medical devices

According to the Medical Devices Directive (93/42/EEC), a medical device is defined as any instrument, apparatus, appliance, material, or other article, whether used alone or in combination, including the software necessary for its proper application intended by the manufacturer to be used for human beings for the purpose of:

- Diagnosis, prevention, monitoring, treatment or alleviation of disease.
- Diagnosis, monitoring, treatment, alleviation of or compensation for an injury or handicap.
- Investigation, replacement, or modification of the anatomy or of a physiological process.
- Control of conception.
- Does not achieve its principal intended action in or on the human body by pharmacological, immunological, or metabolic means, but which may be assisted in its function by such means.

Medical devices are classified according to a risk-based approach; Class I, Class IIa, Class IIb, and Class III, with Class III covering the highest risk products. The classification depends upon the degree of invasiveness, the duration of contact with the body, and the target anatomy.

Device regulation

The regulation covering medical devices is Council Directive 93/42/EEC. The Directive applies to medical devices and their accessories. An accessory, whilst not being a device, is intended specifically by the manufacturer to be used together with a device. Directive 93/42/EEC does not apply to the following products:

- In vitro diagnostic (IVDs) devices that are covered by Directive 98/79/EEC.
- Active implantable devices that are covered by Directive 90/385/EEC.
- Medicinal products that are covered by Directive 2001/83/EC.

In 2012 the EC published proposals for two new Regulations on medical devices and IVDs, which will replace the existing three Directives. The responsibility for ensuring that a product conforms to devices regulation falls to the manufacturer, and compliance with the regulations may involve a review of quality and technical documentation by a notified body (an independent technical testing organization). Notified bodies are designated by competent authorities. A CE mark (use of initials 'CE') is placed on products as a statement of compliance with the essential requirements of the regulation following conformity assessment. A CE marked product can be freely marketed anywhere in the EU without further control. The European Commission's MEDDEVs guidelines aim to promote a common approach in the conformity assessment process.

Essential requirements of devices

Devices must meet certain essential general requirements (set out in Annex I of Directive 93/42/EEC):

- Devices must be designed and manufactured in such a way that, when used under the conditions and for the purposes intended, they will not compromise the clinical condition or the safety of patients, or users.
- The design and construction of the device must conform to safety principles.
- Devices must achieve the performances intended by the manufacturer.
- The characteristics and performance must not be adversely affected during the lifetime of the device, when the device is subjected to the stresses that can occur during normal conditions of use.
- A device must be designed, manufactured, and packed in such a way that their characteristics and performances during their intended use will not be adversely affected during transport and storage.
- Any undesirable side effect must constitute an acceptable risk when weighed against the intended performance.

Borderline products

Borderline products are those that are not easily classified as either a medicinal product or a medical device. If a product acts pharmacologically, metabolically, or immunologically, it is likely to be considered to be a medicinal product. The EC publishes a guidance document that provides explanations of how the determination of a borderline product should be undertaken (MEDDEV 2.1/3).

Instructions for use (IFU)

IFU provide information from the manufacturer, to inform the user of the device of its safe and proper use, its expected performance, and of any precautions to be taken.

Further reading

🔖 http://ec.europa.eu/health/medical-devices/documents/guidelines/index_en.htm

Clinical trials regulation

Clinical Trials Directive (2001/20/EC)

All clinical trials conducted within Europe must comply with the requirements of the Clinical Trials Directive (2001/20/EC). The Directive standardizes the process for regulatory approval of clinical trials, and Article 2 defines a clinical trial as:

> any investigation in human subjects intended to discover or verify the clinical, pharmacological and/or other pharmacodynamic effects of one or more investigational medicinal product(s), and/or to identify adverse reactions to one or more investigational medicinal product(s) and/or to study absorption, distribution, metabolism and excretion of one or more investigational medicinal product(s) with the object of ascertaining its (their) safety and/or efficacy.

The Directive does not apply to non-interventional trials. These are studies where the medicinal product is prescribed in the usual manner in accordance with the terms of the marketing authorization. The Directive is currently under review and consultation by the EC (2012). A proposed Regulation will replace the Directive, ensuring rules for conducting clinical trials are identical throughout the EU (expected to come into effect in 2016).

Sponsor

A sponsor is defined as an individual, company, institution, or organization that takes responsibility for the initiation, management, and/or financing of a clinical trial. A sponsor does not need to be located in a member state, but must have legal representation in the EU. The sponsor may delegate study related duties and delegated duties must be specified in writing. The sponsor remains ultimately responsible for ensuring the conduct of the trial.

Sponsors are responsible for designing, conducting, recording, and reporting clinical studies in accordance with good clinical practice (GCP) principles and standards, ensuring the safety, well-being and rights of clinical trial subjects. Failure to comply with the legislation can result in penalties that include fines and/or a custodial sentence.

Key features of the Directive

- Provides a framework of how clinical trials must be conducted.
- Promotes standardization and harmonization of clinical trial procedures.
- Includes the requirement to carry out all clinical trials in accordance with the principles of GCP, ensuring high standards and minimizing risk to study subjects.
- Clinical trials must have an identified sponsor who takes responsibility for the study.

- The investigational medicinal product (IMP) should be manufactured to GMP standards. An IMP is a pharmaceutical form of an active substance or placebo being tested or used as a reference in a clinical trial.
- Formalizes the protection of patients who are incapable of giving informed consent/minors.
- Provision for GCP and GMP inspection and enforcement powers, improving and ensuring the overall quality of clinical trials.
- Pharmacovigilance arrangements including recording and reporting of serious unexpected serious adverse reactions.

Clinical trial authorization application

A clinical trial may only be undertaken if certain criteria are fulfilled, including gaining ethical and competent authority approval. Importantly, the approval must ensure that the anticipated benefits justify the predicted risks.

The competent authorities assess the clinical trial application (CTA) submitted by sponsors. The submission should detail all the important features of the product, the formulation, toxicology, non-clinical data, and the study protocol. In the UK, CTA forms for initial applications can be completed and downloaded from the Integrated Research Application System (IRAS) website or the European Clinical Trials (EudraCT) website. Authorization by a competent authority should be carried out as rapidly as possible, but must not exceed 60 days.

The sponsor may make changes to the protocol after the study has started for non-substantial amendments. The sponsor must inform the competent authorities if the amendment is considered to be substantial. Amendments are regarded as 'substantial' if they are likely to have a significant impact on the safety, physical or mental integrity of the clinical trial participants or the scientific value of the trial.

First-in-man studies

For first-in-man studies, sponsors are encouraged to identify particular areas of risk and apply risk avoidance strategies wherever possible and/or to seek pre-submission advice. For some novel compounds, where, for example, the mode of action involves multiple signalling pathways or where the compound directly or indirectly affects the immune system, additional expert advice may be sort by the competent authority before authorization.

Further reading

℘ http://www.ec.europa.eu/health/human-use/clinical-trials/index_en.htm#rlctd
℘ https://eudract.ema.europa.eu/
℘ http://www.ema.europa.eu/pdfs/human/swp/2836707enfin.pdf
℘ https://www.myresearchproject.org.uk/

Chapter 2.13

Good clinical practice

Good clinical practice

GCP is a set of internationally recognized ethical and scientific quality standards concerning the designing, conducting, recording, and reporting of clinical trials that involve human subjects. Compliance with GCP principles provides an assurance that the rights, safety, and welfare of trial subjects are protected, and from a regulatory perspective, that the results of the clinical trials are trustworthy and credible.

The principles of GCP are outlined in the GCP Directive 2005/28/EC, the Clinical Trials Directive 2001/20/EC, and the ICH guideline on GCP ICH Topic E6. ICH E6 covers important definitions, ethical committee review, the role of the investigator and sponsor, the expect contents of the clinical trial protocol, and investigator's brochure. The topic provides a unified standard for the EU, USA, and Japan, facilitating the mutual acceptance of clinical data by regulatory authorities. Practical advice about implementing the principles of GCP can be found in the MHRA's Good Clinical Practice Guide.

Core good clinical practice principles

The core ICH GCP principles are:
- Clinical trials should be conducted in accordance with the ethical principles that have their origin in the Declaration of Helsinki.
- A trial should only be initiated and continued if the anticipated benefits justify the risks.
- The rights, safety, and well-being of trial subjects are the most important considerations, and should prevail over interests of science and society.
- The available non-clinical and clinical information on an investigational product should be adequate to support the proposed clinical trial.
- Clinical trials should be scientifically sound and be clearly described in a detailed protocol.
- A trial should be conducted in compliance with the protocol that has received prior Institutional Review Board (IRB)/Independent Ethics Committee (IEC) approval.
- The medical care given to, and medical decisions made on behalf of, subjects should always be the responsibility of a qualified physician.
- Individuals involved in conducting a trial should be qualified by education, training, and experience to perform his or her respective tasks.
- Freely-given informed consent should be obtained from every subject prior to clinical trial participation.
- All clinical trial information should be recorded, handled, and stored in a way that allows its accurate reporting, interpretation and verification.
- The confidentiality of records that could identify subjects should be protected, respecting the privacy and confidentiality rules.
- Investigational products should be manufactured, handled, and stored in accordance with applicable good manufacturing practice (GMP) and used in accordance with the approved protocol.
- Systems with procedures that assure the quality of every aspect of the trial should be implemented.

Good clinical practice inspection

A clinical trial sponsor is the individual or organization which takes responsibility for the initiation, conduct, and management of the trial. The sponsor must ensure that the trial is conducted according to the principles of GCP and that investigators are adequately informed and suitably qualified. The trial investigator, the individual who directly administers the investigational product to the study subject, must perform their duties in compliance with GCP principles and must clearly document when trial related duties have been delegated to others.

GCP inspectors assess compliance with the requirements of the legislation and guidelines relating to the conduct of clinical trials involving investigational medicinal products. In the UK, the MHRA inspectorate is responsible for inspecting clinical trials for compliance with GCP. Inspection sites may include pharmaceutical companies, contract research organizations, and non-commercial organizations such as universities.

There are three types of GCP inspection in the UK:
* Routine inspections: organizations are notified of the inspection in advance.
* Triggered inspections: these *ad hoc* inspections are triggered by suspected violations of the legislation relating to the conduct of clinical trials, and in rare circumstances the organization may not be notified in advance.
* CHMP requested inspections: the CHMP can request GCP inspections in relation to marketing authorization applications made using the EU Centralized Procedure. EMA co-ordinated inspections are conducted by inspectors from EU MSs.

Further reading

🕮 http://www.ich.org/
🕮 http://www.ema.europa.eu/pdfs/human/ich/013595en.pdf
🕮 http://www.mhra.gov.uk/Howweregulate/Medicines/Inspectionandstandards/GoodClinicalPractice/index.htm and the Good Clinical Practice Guide
🕮 http://www.ema.europa.eu/Inspections/GCPgeneral.html

Good laboratory practice and good clinical laboratory practice

Good laboratory practice

GLP embodies a set of principles that provides a framework of standards within which laboratory studies are planned, performed, monitored, recorded, reported and archived. The principles of GLP help promote the collection of high quality data and reduce the need for duplicate testing. Broadly, GLP principles specifically cover the following themes:

- Test facility organization and personnel.
- Quality assurance programme.
- Laboratory facilities.
- Apparatus, material, and reagents.
- Test systems.
- Test and reference substances.
- Standard operating procedures.
- Performance of the study.
- Reporting of study results.
- Storage and retention of records and material.

Organization for Economic Co-operation and Development

In 1981 the Organization for Economic Co-operation and Development (OECD) finalized agreed principles of GLP. This led to the OECD Council's decision on the Mutual Acceptance of Data (MAD) (see Box 2.14.1).

Box 2.14.1 MAD decision of the OECD Council

Data generated in the testing of chemicals in an OECD member country in accordance with OECD Test Guidelines and OECD Principles of Good Laboratory Practice shall be accepted in other member countries for purposes of assessment and other uses relating to the protection of man and the environment.

Reproduced from the OECD, 'Decision of the Council concerning the Mutual Acceptance of Data in the Assessment of Chemicals', 12 May 1981—C(81)30/FINAL Amended on 26 November 1997—C(97)186/FINAL. Available at: ✍ http://acts.oecd.org

In 1983 the OECD recommended that implementation of GLP compliance should be verified by study audits and laboratory inspections.

Regulation

In the EU, Council Directives 2004/9/EC and 2004/10/EC concern the application of the principles, inspection, and verification of GLP. This is a regulatory requirement that helps reassure the regulatory authorities that the data submitted are a true reflection of the results and the data can be confidently relied upon when making risk benefit decisions. Research not conducted according to GLP principles is generally not included in the regulatory review of marketing authorization applications. For biopharmaceuticals, however, it is recognized that some studies employing specialized test systems may not be able to comply fully with GLP (ICH S 6 Preclinical Safety Evaluation of Biotechnology-derived Pharmaceuticals). Facilities that conduct regulatory studies are subject to GLP compliance and can be assessed and monitored through inspection. A 'regulatory study' is defined as a non-clinical experiment or set of experiments:

• In which an item is examined under laboratory conditions or in the environment in order to obtain data on its properties or its safety (or both) with respect to human health.
• The results of which are for, or intended for, submission to the appropriate regulatory authorities.
• Compliance with the principles of GLP is required in respect of that experiment or set of experiments by the appropriate regulatory authorities.

Good clinical laboratory practice

The principles of GLP have been applied to the analysis of clinical samples in a relatively new concept termed good clinical laboratory practice (GCLP). GCLP provides an appropriate standard for sample analysis within clinical studies. Like GLP, GCLP defines a broad range of principles. These principles include the roles and responsibilities of laboratory staff, facilities for archiving, standard operating procedures (SOPs), reporting results, conduct of work, and confidentiality.

Further reading

Ezzelle J, Rodriguez-Chavez IR, Darden JM, et al. (2008). Guidelines on good clinical laboratory practice: bridging operations between research and clinical research laboratories. *J Pharm Biomed Anal* **46**(1), 18–29.

⚲ http://www.ich.org/
⚲ http://www.ema.europa.eu/Inspections/GLP.html
⚲ http://www.mhra.gov.uk/Howweregulate/Medicines/Inspectionandstandards/GoodLaboratory Practice/index.htm
⚲ http://www.oecd.org/env/ehs/risk-assessment/oecdinstrumentsforensuringmutualacceptanceofdata. htm

Chapter 2.15

Good manufacturing practice

Quality assurance

Quality Assurance (QA) is a concept that covers all matters influencing the quality of a product. The EU definition of GMP according to European Commission Directive 2003/94/EC is 'the part of quality assurance which ensures that products are consistently produced and controlled in accordance with the quality standards appropriate to their intended use'.

Good manufacturing practice

Within the EU, a system of marketing authorizations exists to ensure that all medicinal products are assessed in relation to quality, safety and efficacy. Similarly, a system of manufacturing authorizations ensures that all manufacturers of medicinal products hold a valid manufacturing authorization. The issue of a manufacturing authorization is dependent upon regular satisfactory inspection by a relevant competent authority, generally on a 3-yearly basis.

The principles and guidelines of GMP for medicinal products for human use and investigational medicinal products for human use are laid down in EC Directive 2003/94/EC. From a practical perspective, the principles of GMP apply to any manufacturing operations for medicinal products that require authorizations under Article 40 of Directive 2001/83/EC, Article 44 of Directive 2001/82/EC or Article 13 of Directive 2001/20/EC (as amended). In order for a manufacturer to gain and hold a manufacturing authorization, it must demonstrate that it manufactures products in compliance with the principles and guidelines of GMP and in accordance with any manufacturing and marketing authorizations held.

Inspection

During regular inspection, inspectors will examine the quality system in place at the site of manufacture. Such a system is designed to ensure that a product is manufactured to the required quality for its intended use. This quality system must include regular periodic or rolling reviews of licensed products manufactured at the site to verify consistency of the processes and identify areas for improvement.

Standards and guidance

Although the principles of GMP include many of the aspects of the International Standard for Quality Management Systems (ISO 9001:2000) and the standards of the European Committee for Standardization (CEN), these standards are not used to govern the production and the quality control of medicinal products, for which the principles and guidelines of GMP are applied.

Guidance on the interpretation of the principles and guidelines of good manufacturing practices for medicinal products for human and veterinary use laid down in the aforementioned Directives is published in *EudraLex—Volume 4* of *The Rules Governing Medicinal Products in the European Union*. This guidance is used in the assessment of applications for marketing authorization applications for medicinal products and also forms a basis for the inspection of manufacturers of medicinal products.

Volume 4 of EudraLex is also known as the 'EU guide to GMP' and consists of three parts and numerous annexes:
- Part I includes guidance for the basic requirements for medicinal products.
- Part II includes guidance for active substances used as starting materials for medicinal products.
- Part III consists of GMP-related documents, including clarification on regulatory expectations and information on best practice.
- Annexes contain guidance on specific areas of manufacture, including the manufacture of sterile medicinal products, radiopharmaceuticals, herbal medicinal products, products derived from human blood or blood plasma, and parametric release.

National guides to GMP exist in the EU, such as the *Rules and Guidance for Pharmaceutical Manufacturers and Distributors* in the UK (commonly known as 'The Orange Guide'). All updates to the EU guide to GMP are reproduced in the UK Orange Guide.

Further reading
 http://ec.europa.eu/health/documents/eudralex/vol-4/index_en.htm

The Ethics Committee (EU)

Overview

An Ethics Committee (EthC) is an independent body in a member state (MS), consisting of healthcare professionals and non-medical members, whose responsibility it is to protect the rights, safety, and well-being of human subjects involved in a trial and to provide public assurance of that protection.

Considerations of the Ethics Committee

In preparing its opinion, the EthC shall consider, in particular:
- The relevance of the clinical trial and the trial design.
- Whether the evaluation of the anticipated benefits and risks as required under Directive 2001/20/EC Article 3(2)(a) is satisfactory.
- The protocol.
- The suitability of the investigator and supporting staff.
- The investigator's brochure.
- The quality of the facilities.
- The adequacy and completeness of the written information to be given and the procedure to be followed for the purpose of obtaining informed consent and the justification for the research on persons incapable of giving informed consent as regards the specific restrictions laid down in Article 3.
- Provision for indemnity or compensation.
- Any insurance or indemnity to cover the liability of the investigator and sponsor.
- The amounts and, where appropriate, the arrangements for rewarding or compensating investigators and trial subjects and the relevant aspects of any agreement between the sponsor and the site.
- The arrangements for the recruitment of subjects.

A clinical trial may be initiated only if the EthC and/or the competent authority comes to the conclusion that the anticipated therapeutic and public health benefits justify the risks, and may be continued only if compliance with this requirement is permanently monitored.

Membership

A typical research EthC meets once a month. A committee usually has 12–18 members, which should have the following membership:

- The chairman.
- Vice-chairman and alternate vice-chairman.
- Expert members.
- One-third of the members should be lay persons. Half of those should have no connection with health and social care.
- Someone with knowledge of statistics.
- Both sexes, a range of ages, and a range of ethnic minorities should be represented.

The tenure of appointment will be 3–5 years, renewable for a further term. In addition, the committee must appoint a mentor. The quorum necessary to hold a legitimate meeting is 7 members, and it must include the chairman, vice-chairman or an alternate vice-chairman, one lay member, and one expert member.

Timelines for review

The EthC has a maximum of 60 days from the date of receipt of a valid application to give its opinion. Within this period the EthC may send a single request for information supplementary to that already supplied by the applicant. No extension to the 60-day period is permissible except in the case of trials involving medicinal products for gene therapy or somatic cell therapy or medicinal products containing genetically-modified organisms. In this case, an extension of a maximum of 30 days shall be permitted. For these products, this 90-day period may be extended by a further 90 days in the event of consultation of a group or a committee. In the case of xenogenic cell therapy, there shall be no time limit to the authorization period.

Multi-centre trials

For multi-centre clinical trials limited to a single country, a procedure exists to provide a single EthC opinion for that country. In the case of multi-centre clinical trials carried out in more than one country simultaneously, a single opinion shall be given for each country concerned by the clinical trial.

In the UK, all clinical trials involving human subjects and the testing of IMPs require approval from a United Kingdom Ethics Committee Authority (UKECA) recognized Research Ethics Committee REC. Any recognized Multi-centre Research Ethics Committee (MREC) or Local Research Ethics Committee (LREC) can consider multi-site research and their decisions will be nationally binding.

Single-site research can be considered by a recognized or authorized LREC in the domain or the neighbouring domain in which the research chief investigator is professionally based.

Further reading

Directive 2001/20/EC of the European Parliament and of the Council of 4th April 2001. Available at:
    http://www.eortc.be/services/doc/clinical-eu-directive-04-april-01.pdf

The Institutional Review Board (US)

Overview

An IRB, also known as an Independent Ethics Committee (IEC) or Ethical Review Board (ERB), is a committee that has been formally designated to approve, monitor, and review biomedical and behavioural research involving humans with the aim to protect the rights and welfare of the research subjects.

In the United States, IRBs are governed by Title 45 CFR, Part 46.

Considerations of the Ethics Committee

The purpose of an IRB review is to assure, both in advance and by periodic review, that appropriate steps are taken to protect the rights and welfare of humans participating as subjects in a research study. Special attention should be paid to trials that may include vulnerable subjects, such as pregnant women, children, prisoners, the elderly, or persons with diminished comprehension. The IRB/IEC should review the following documents:
- Trial protocol/amendments.
- Written informed consent form(s) and consent form updates that the investigator proposes for use in the trial.
- Subject recruitment procedures (e.g. advertisements).
- Written information to be provided to subjects.
- Investigator's brochure (IB).
- Available safety information.
- Information about payments and compensation available to subjects.
- Investigator's current curriculum vitae and/or other documentation evidencing qualifications.
- Any other documents that the IRB/IEC may need to fulfil its responsibilities.

Timelines for review

The IRB/IEC should review a proposed clinical trial within a reasonable time. The timelines vary depending on the type of study. Exempt studies (posing minimal risk to human subjects) are approved in 2–3 weeks from receipt. Expedited studies take 3–4 weeks. The IRB/IEC must document its views in writing, clearly identifying the trial, the documents reviewed, and the dates for the following:
- Approval/favourable opinion.
- Modifications required prior to its approval/favourable opinion.
- Disapproval/negative opinion.
- Termination/suspension of any prior approval/favourable opinion.

Membership of the Institutional Review Board

The composition of an IRB for the FDA's requirements is set in 21 CFR 56.107.

- The IRB must have at least five members.
- The members must have enough experience, expertise, and diversity to make an informed decision on whether the research is ethical, informed consent is sufficient, and appropriate safeguards have been put in place.
- The IRB should include both men and women, as long as they aren't chosen specifically for their gender.
- The members of the IRB must not be all of the same profession.
- The IRB must include at least one scientist and at least one non-scientist.
- The IRB must include at least one 'community member', a person who is not affiliated with the institution or in the immediate family of a person affiliated with the institution.
- IRB members may not vote on their own projects.
- The IRB may include consultants in their discussions to meet requirements for expertise or diversity, but only actual IRB members may vote.

In order to vote on a proposal, more than half of the members of the board must be present and there must be a non-scientist present. There are exceptions for expedited review, where only the chair of the committee or a designee reviews research, but these are relatively narrow.

Further reading

Code of Federal Regulations (2005). Title 45, Part 46, Protection of Human Subjects, June 23.
Code of Federal Regulations (2012). Title 21, Volume 1. Revised as of April 1.

Chapter 2.18

Marketing authorization applications and updating and maintaining licences

Marketing authorization applications (MAAs)

According to Article 6 of Directive 2001/83/EC, no medicinal product may be placed on the market of a member state unless a marketing authorization has been issued. In order to gain an authorization, an MAA must be submitted to the competent authority. An MAA consists of a body of evidence submitted as a dossier. All applications must be submitted in the CTD format and the dossier of information in support of the MAA is organized into five separate modules:

• Module 1 (administrative details, including the product literature).
• Module 2 (expert summaries providing an overview of the quality, non-clinical, and clinical components of the application).
• Module 3 (quality data).
• Module 4 (non-clinical data).
• Module 5 (clinical data).

Most MAAs are submitted to competent authorities by the pharmaceutical industry, although institutions with the obligatory supporting data may apply. MAAs are assessed by multidisciplinary teams of scientific, pharmaceutical, and medical assessors, who weigh up the risk benefit of the proposed product. For approval, the evaluation by the competent authority must objectively conclude that the new medicinal product has acceptable quality, safety and efficacy, in line with current standards and regulatory guidance. Accordingly, Article 26 of Directive 2001/83/EC states that a marketing authorization can be refused if the benefit risk balance is not considered favourable or if therapeutic efficacy is insufficiently substantiated.

Specials

Exemptions to the provision of an MAA are detailed in Article 5 of Directive 2001/83/EC, where, in order to fulfil special needs, a medicinal product may be supplied without a marketing authorization in response to a *bona fide* unsolicited order, formulated in accordance with the specifications of an authorized healthcare professional and for use by an individual patient under his direct personal responsibility.

Legal basis

The legal basis of an MAA depends on the active ingredient of the medicinal product, and the majority of MAAs concern medicinal products with well-known active substances. Such medicinal products can be submitted as abridged applications, where applicants do not necessarily have to repeat non-clinical and clinical testing. Applications submitted under Article 10 of Directive 2001/83/EC describe generic applications (Article 10(1)), well established use (Article 10a), fixed combination (Article 10b), and informed consent applications (Article 10c). Applications submitted under Article 8(3) must be accompanied by pharmaceutical tests, non-clinical tests, and clinical trials.

Maintaining a marketing authorization

A marketing authorization is held by a marketing authorization holder (MAH), and following approval are generally valid for 5 years. Marketing authorizations are renewed by the competent authority and renewals should be submitted at least 6 months prior to expiry. Once renewed, the marketing authorization is generally valid for the commercial life of the product, unless there are potential ongoing safety concerns. In such circumstances, the renewal would be for other 5 years. If a MAH does not wish to renew the licence, the competent authority should be informed in writing by submitting a cancellation letter.

Article 23a of Directive 2001/83/EC refers to the statutory requirement of the MAH to inform the licensing authority of any disruptions to the supply of the medicine. The MAH is required to inform the competent authority of the date of actual marketing of the medicinal product and to inform the competent authority if the product ceases to be placed on the market either temporarily or permanently. The so-called Sunset clause states that the marketing authorization will cease to be valid if the medicinal product is not placed on the market within 3 years of the authorization or where a medicinal product previously placed on the market is no longer actually present on the market for three consecutive years.

Changes to a marketing authorization

Changes to marketing authorizations are necessary so that the product licence can be kept up to date and so the product literature adequately reflects current scientific developments, evolving safety profiles and advances in clinical practice. Such changes to an MA are agreed with a competent authority by a variation application. Depending on the complexity of the proposed change, variation applications include Type IA, Type IB and Type II (Directive 1234/2008).

Further reading

🔗 http://www.mhra.gov.uk/Howweregulate/Medicines/index.htm
🔗 http://www.ema.europa.eu/htms/human/raguidelines/pre.htm

The International Conference on Harmonisation

The International Conference on Harmonisation (ICH)

The ICH of Technical Requirements for Registration of Pharmaceuticals for Human Use brings together representatives from regulatory authorities and pharmaceutical industry associations in Europe, Japan, and the USA. The initiative involves regulators and industry as equal partners.

ICH is operated via the ICH steering committee, which is supported by ICH co-ordinators and the ICH Secretariat. Working within the ICH terms of reference, the steering committee selects topics for harmonization, determines the policies and procedures for ICH, and monitors progress in harmonization.

The ICH steering committee comprises of six 'directly involved parties' (the founder members of ICH), three 'observers', and the International Federation of Pharmaceutical Manufacturers & Associations (IFPMA), who host the ICH secretariat.

The six members are:
- The EU.
- European Federation of Pharmaceutical Industries and Associations (EFPIA).
- MHLW, Japan.
- Japan Pharmaceutical Manufacturers Association (JPMA).
- US FDA.
- Pharmaceutical Research and Manufacturers of America (PhRMA).

The three observers are:
- The World Health Organization (WHO).
- The EFTA.
- Canada (represented by Health Canada).

Objectives of the ICH

The purpose and objectives of ICH are:
- To discuss scientific and technical aspects of medicinal product registration.
- To make recommendations on ways of achieving harmonization in the interpretation and application of technical guidelines and requirements for medicinal product registration.
- To reduce or obviate the need for duplicate testing when developing new medicinal products.
- To foster more economical use of human, animal, and material resources.
- To eliminate as much as possible unnecessary delay in the global development and availability of new medicinal products whilst safeguarding quality, safety, and efficacy.

ICH topics

ICH topics are divided into four major categories, which are assigned 'Codes':

- Quality topics are designated by Q. These relate to chemical and pharmaceutical quality assurance and examples include:
  - Q3A—Impurities in New Drug Substances;
  - Q3B—Impurities in New Drug Products;
  - Q3C—Impurities: Guideline for Residual Solvents.
- Safety topics are designated by S. These relate to in vitro and in vivo non-clinical studies and examples include:
  - S1A—Need of Carcinogenicity Studies of Pharmaceuticals;
  - S1B—Testing for Carcinogenicity of Pharmaceuticals;
  - S1C—Dose Selection for Carcinogenicity Studies of Pharmaceuticals.
- Efficacy topics are designated by E. These relate to clinical studies in human subjects, and include both efficacy and safety. Examples include:
  - E8—General Consideration of Clinical Trials;
  - E9—Statistical Principles for Clinical Trials;
  - E10—Choice of Control Group and Related Issues in Clinical Trials.
- Multidisciplinary topics are designated by M. These are cross-cutting topics that do not fit into one of the above categories and examples include:
  - M1—MedDRA Medical Dictionary for Regulatory Activities;
  - M4—CTD The Common Technical Document.

Modifications to ICH guidelines are designated as (R1), (R2), (R3), etc., depending on the revision.

Further reading

℘ http://www.ich.org

Chapter 2.20

Common technical document

Overview

The common technical document (CTD) is a format agreed upon by ICH to organize applications to regulatory authorities for registration of pharmaceuticals for human use. Each region has had its own requirements for the organization of the technical reports in the submission and for the preparation of the summaries and tables. In Japan, the applicants prepared the GAIYO. In Europe, expert reports and tabulated summaries were required, and written summaries were recommended. The US FDA had guidance regarding the format and content of the NDA. To avoid the need to generate and compile different registration dossiers, a guideline was developed by the EMA, the US FDA, and the MHLW Japan, to create a format for the CTD that would be acceptable in all three regions. All three parties accepted applications in this format from 1 July 2001.

Content

The CTD is divided into 5 modules (see Fig. 2.20.1):
- Administrative and prescribing information.
- Overview and summary of the data submitted in modules 3–5.
- Quality (pharmaceutical documentation).
- Safety (non-clinical toxicology studies).
- Pharmacology, efficacy, and safety (clinical studies).

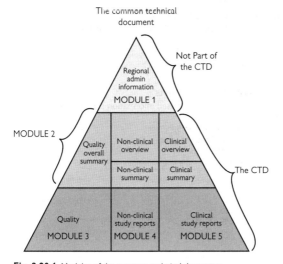

Fig. 2.20.1 Modules of the common technical document.

Module 1: administrative information and prescribing information

- This module should contain region specific documentation.
- The content and format of this module can be specified by the relevant regulatory authorities.

Module 2: common technical document summaries

Module 2 should begin with a general introduction to the pharmaceutical, including its pharmacological class, mode of action, and proposed clinical use. Module 2 should contain 7 sections:

- CTD Table of contents.
- CTD Introduction.
- Quality overall summary.
- Non-clinical overview.
- Clinical overview.
- Non-clinical written and tabulated summaries.
- Clinical summary.

Module 3: quality

This section provides guidance on the format of a registration application for drug substances and drug products. The content should include relevant information described in existing ICH guidance. It is organized as follows:

- Table of contents of Module 3.
- Body of data.
- Literature references.

Module 4: non-clinical study reports

The non-clinical study reports should be presented in the order described below:

- Table of contents of Module 4.
- Study reports.
- Literature references.

Module 5: clinical study reports

The human study reports and related information should be presented in the order described:

- Table of contents of Module 5.
- Tabular listing of all clinical studies.
- Clinical study reports.
- Literature references.

Benefits

There are a number of benefits to both applicant and reviewer in having this common format, as outlined below:

- More user-friendly documentation.
- Shortens review time.
- Saves resources.
- Facilitates exchange of information and discussion.
- More consistent reviews.

Further reading

ICH Topic M4, Common technical document for the registration of pharmaceuticals for human use—organization of CTD. Available at: ℘ http://www.ich.org/

Medicinal product information in the European Union

Summary of product characteristics

The summary of product characteristics (SmPC) is a source of information for healthcare professionals on how to administer a medicinal product safely and effectively. Its content also forms the basis for any subsequent advertising claims. The SmPC does not normally give general recommendations concerning the treatment of a particular medical condition. According to Directive 2001/83/EC and Regulation (EC) 726/2004, a SmPC must be included with an MAA. The SmPC forms an intrinsic and essential part of an MAA, and reflects the characteristics of the medicinal product agreed during the course of the licensing procedure. The SmPC is divided into a number of sections. These include:

- Qualitative and quantitative composition (Section 2).
- Pharmaceutical form (Section 3).
- Clinical particulars, such as the indications and posology, warnings, and side effects (Section 4).
- Pharmacological properties (Section 5).
- Pharmaceutical particulars (Section 6).

Each section details issues that relate to the core population, followed by information on special populations, where appropriate (paediatrics, elderly, or renal and hepatic impairment). Consistent medical terminology is used throughout (Medical Dictionary for Regulatory Activities [MedDRA]). The content of a marketed SmPC can only be changed after agreement and approval from a competent authority.

Package leaflet

Directive 2001/83/EC defines a package leaflet (PL) as a leaflet containing information for the user which accompanies the medicinal product, and all medicines are required by European law to be accompanied by a PL. The PL is also sometimes referred to as the patient information leaflet or PIL. Article 59(1) of Directive 2001/83/EC requires that the PL be consistent with the information contained in the SmPC, and a draft package leaflet should be submitted to the competent authority at the time of an MAA. The PL is divided into sections, including:

- What the product is.
- Before you take the product.
- How to take the product.
- Potential side effects.
- Storage instructions.

Readability

The PL should contain comprehensive information that is understandable and easily accessible. It is therefore important that the PL is clearly worded so that patients can use their medicine successfully. In order to confirm readability of the PL, Article 59(3) of Directive 2001/83/EC states that the PL should reflect the results of user testing with target patient groups to ensure that it is easy to use and understandable. It is a requirement for marketing authorization that the results of such consultations are provided to a competent authority for assessment.

Labelling

The immediate packaging is the container or other form of packaging immediately in contact with the medicinal product. The outer packaging is the packaging into which is placed the immediate packaging. The labelling is the information on the immediate and outer packaging. Appropriate labelling is essential for the safe use of medicines. Labels should be unambiguous and allowing easy identification of the product, minimizing risk of administration error. Article 56a of Directive 2001/83/EC requires the name of the medicinal product to be expressed in Braille format on the packaging.

Guidelines

The quality review of document (QRD) template sets out standard headings and defines the format for product information for medicinal products. Further specific guidance is provided in the *Rules Governing Medicinal Products in the European Union*, Volume 2C, *Notice to Applicants*.

Further reading

℘ http://www.ema.europa.eu/htms/human/qrd/qrdintro.htm
℘ http://ec.europa.eu/enterprise/sectors/pharmaceuticals/documents/eudralex/vol-2/index_en.htm
℘ http://www.mhra.gov.uk/Howweregulate/Medicines/Labelspatientinformationleafletsandpackaging/index.htm

Summary of product characteristics

Overview

The summary of product characteristics (SmPC) is a specific document required within the EC before any medicinal product is authorized for marketing. Article 8(3)(j) of Directive 2001/83/EC and Article 6(1) of Regulation (EC) 726/2004 require that, in order to obtain a MA, a SmPC in accordance with Article 11 of Directive 2001/83/EC must be included in the application.

This summary sets out the agreed position of the medicinal product as distilled during the course of the assessment process. It is therefore the definitive description of the product both in terms of its properties—chemical, pharmacological, and pharmaceutical—and the clinical use to which it can put. As such, the content cannot be changed except with the approval of the originating competent authority. When updated pharmacovigilance data are considered to impact on the risk-benefit profile of the medicinal product, the competent authority (CA) may request a variation to the SmPC.

The SmPC is the basis of information for health professionals on how to use the medicinal product safely and effectively. The PL shall be drawn up in accordance with the SmPC. The Guideline on excipients in the label and Package leaflet of medicinal products for human use is also applicable to the SmPC.

Separate SmPCs are required for each pharmaceutical form and strength by the EC and certain MSs. For the purposes of giving information to prescribers, the SmPCs of different pharmaceutical forms and strengths may be combined for appropriate products within the same range.

Contents

The summary of the product characteristics shall contain, in the order indicated below, the following sections:
1. Name of the medicinal product followed by the strength and the pharmaceutical form.
2. Qualitative and quantitative composition in terms of the active substances and constituents of the excipient, knowledge of which is essential for proper administration of the medicinal product. The usual common name or chemical description shall be used.
3. Pharmaceutical form.
4. Clinical particulars:
     4.1—therapeutic indications;
     4.2—posology and method of administration for adults and, where necessary, for children;
     4.3—contra-indications;
     4.4—special warnings and precautions for use and, in the case of immunological medicinal products, any special precautions to be taken by persons handling such products and administering them to patients, together with any precautions to be taken by the patient;
     4.5—interaction with other medicinal products and other forms of interactions;

4.6—use during pregnancy and lactation;
4.7—effects on ability to drive and to use machines;
4.8—undesirable effects;
4.9—overdose (symptoms, emergency procedures, antidotes).
5. Pharmacological properties:
   5.1—pharmacodynamic properties;
   5.2—pharmacokinetic properties;
   5.3—preclinical safety data.
6. Pharmaceutical particulars:
   6.1—list of excipients;
   6.2—major incompatibilities;
   6.3—shelf life, when necessary after reconstitution of the medicinal product or when the immediate packaging is opened for the first time;
   6.4—special precautions for storage;
   6.5—nature and contents of container;
   6.6—special precautions for disposal of a used medicinal product or waste materials derived from such medicinal product, if appropriate.
7. Marketing authorization holder.
8. Marketing authorization number(s).
9. Date of the first authorization or renewal of the authorization.
10. Date of revision of the text.
11. Dosimetry for radiopharmaceuticals, full details of internal radiation.
12. For radiopharmaceuticals, additional detailed instructions for preparation and quality control of such preparation and, where appropriate, maximum storage times.

Further reading

European Commission. Volume 2C *Notice to Applicants. A guideline on summary of product characteristics (SmPC)* (2009). Available at: ℘ http://ec.europa.eu/health/documents/eudralex/vol-2/index_en.htm

Chapter 2.23

Orphan drugs

Rare diseases

It is estimated that there are between 5000 and 8000 distinct rare diseases. Patients suffering from rare diseases are entitled to the same quality of treatment as other patients with more common diseases. However, some conditions occur so rarely that the cost of developing a drug may not be recovered by the expected sales. In order to encourage development and research, a supportive legislative framework for medicines for rare diseases has been adopted:

- United States in 1983 (the Orphan Drug Act).
- Japan in 1993 (Pharmaceutical Affairs Law amended to incorporate the Orphan Drug Development Support Program).
- Australia in 1998 (Regulation 16J of the Therapeutic Goods Regulations).
- European Union in 2000 (Regulation No 141/2000 and No 847/2000).

Orphan drugs in the European Union

In Europe, applications for designation of orphan medicines are reviewed by the EMA through the COMP. The COMP is responsible for examining applications for orphan designation and adopts a positive or negative opinion on whether the medicinal product should receive orphan status. COMP opinions are ratified by the EC. Sponsors may apply for a designation at any stage in the development of a product, prior to a marketing authorization application. The criteria for orphan designation are found in Regulation 141/2000:

- The product is intended for the diagnosis, prevention, or treatment of a life-threatening or chronically debilitating condition affecting no more than 5 in 10,000 persons in the EU at the time of submission of the designation application (translates into approximately 246,000 persons in the 27 EU member states).

Or,

- The product is intended for the diagnosis, prevention, or treatment of a life-threatening, seriously debilitating or serious and chronic condition and without incentives it is unlikely that expected sales of the medicinal product would cover the investment in its development.

And,

- No satisfactory method of diagnosis, prevention or treatment of the condition concerned is authorized, or, if such method exists, the medicinal product will be of significant benefit to those affected by the condition.

Significant benefit

Significant benefit is defined as a clinically relevant advantage or major contribution to patient care (e.g. better efficacy, safety, administration route). The concept of significant benefit is not considered if there are no available treatment options for the condition.

Incentives

Sponsors that are assigned an orphan designation benefit from incentives:

- A period of 10 years marketing exclusivity, directly competitive similar products cannot normally be placed on the market.
- Protocol assistance in the form of scientific advice to optimize the development of the medicinal product.
- Fee reductions for marketing authorization applications.

Marketing authorization

It is mandatory for all orphan designated medicinal products to use the centralized procedure for marketing authorization applications and such products may be approved under exceptions circumstances. However, Orphan designation does not alter the standard regulatory requirements for obtaining marketing approval, and the safety and efficacy of a product must still be established.

Orphan drugs in the USA

In the United States, the FDA, through its Office of Orphan Products Development (OOPD) administers the major provisions of the Orphan Drug Act. An orphan drug is classified as having a target patient population of <200,000 people in the USA. Incentives include a 7-year period of market exclusivity and tax advantages. A common EMA/FDA application form is available. This can be used for the same medicinal product with the same indication.

Further reading

℞ http://www.emea.europa.eu/htms/human/orphans/guidance.htm
℞ http://www.fda.gov/AboutFDA/CentersOffices/OfficeofMedicalProductsandTobacco/Officeof
    ScienceandHealthCoordination/ucm2018190.htm

Paediatric investigational plans

Overview

A paediatric investigation plan (PIP) is a development plan aimed at ensuring that the necessary data are obtained through studies in children, when it is safe to do so, to support the authorization of a medicine for children. In the EU an agreed PIP must be in place before the adult marketing authorization application is submitted (reviewed by the EMA's PDCO), and in the US paediatric trials are supported by the Best Pharmaceuticals for Children Act.

Both the EU and FDA offer scientific advice procedures which guide clinical trial design to gain a paediatric indication.

The normal development of a medicine requires that various studies be performed to ensure its quality, safety, and efficacy. The development plan are often modified at a later stage, as knowledge increases. Modifications can also be made if difficulties are encountered with delivering the plan, such as around feasibility or as knowledge of the profile of the medicine develops:

- PIPs include a description of the studies and of the measures to adapt the medicine's formulation to make its use more acceptable in children, such as use of a liquid formulation rather than large tablets.
- PIPs cover the needs of all age groups of children, from birth to adolescence, and must include a full description of epidemiology as it applies to the paediatric population.
- PIPs define the timing of studies in children compared to adults, particularly with new classes or for biologicals when little knowledge about the compound is known, the studies may be significantly delayed.

In some cases, studies can be deferred until after the studies in adults have been conducted. This ensures that research in children is done only when it is safe and ethical to do so. Even in this case, however, the PIP should include details of the studies and a timeline.

Some diseases do not affect children (for example, Parkinson's disease), and the development of medicines for these diseases should not be performed in children. In these cases, a PIP is waived.

All applications are reviewed by the EMA centrally; there is no opportunity to submit to a single country.

Templates exist for everything concerning the application, even including the letter of intent to submit, and applications are heard according to a strict timetable.

FDA and EMA are well co-ordinated with respect to paediatric applications, and the links to further information for both the FDA and EMA websites are provided under Further reading.

Further reading

 http://www.ema.europa.eu/ema/index.jsp?curl=pages/regulation/document_listing/document_listing_000293.jsp&mid=WC0b01ac0580025b91&jsenabled=true

 http://www.fda.gov/Drugs/DevelopmentApprovalProcess/DevelopmentResources/ucm049867.htm

Regulatory requirements for pharmacovigilance

Pharmacovigilance

New medicinal products carry unknown risks. Real life drug use cannot be replicated in clinical studies and many adverse reactions will only be detected once a product has been used in large number of the patient. Pharmacovigilance is a risk management process for medicines. Pharmacovigilance is the science and activities relating to the detection, assessment, understanding and prevention of adverse effects or any other drug-related problems. Pharmacovigilance activities include:

• Collecting and managing data on the safety of medicines.
• Reviewing data to detect new or changing safety issues (signals).
• Assessing and evaluating safety data in order to make safety decisions.
• Acting to protect public health.
• Engaging in efficient communication between different stakeholders and people of diverse cultural backgrounds.
• Auditing the outcomes of actions taken and the key processes involved.

Regulation

The Thalidomide disaster of the 1960s stimulated governments into taking action towards assuring the safety of medicinal products and the introduction of more effective drug regulation has resulted in safer medicines. More recently, Regulation (EU) No 1235/2010 (amending, as regards pharmacovigilance of medicinal products for human use, Regulation (EC) No 726/2004) and Directive 2010/84/EU (amending, as regards pharmacovigilance, Directive 2001/83/EC) became applicable in July 2012. The new legislation strengthens the current system for monitoring the safety of medicines. One of the key changes is the establishment of a new EMA committee, the Pharmacovigilance Risk Assessment Committee (PRAC), which can impose on MAH obligations to conduct post-authorization studies (efficacy and safety).

These legal texts are supplemented by Commission Regulation (EEC) 540/95, which concerns suspected unexpected non-serious adverse reactions and the Clinical Trials Directive 2001/20/EC. In addition to the legal texts, detailed information regarding the precise execution of pharmacovigilance related activities are found in ICH guidelines (E2 Topics), the CIOMS Working Group documents (Council for International Organizations of Medical Sciences) and The Guidelines for Pharmacovigilance for Medicinal Products for Human Use (Good Pharmacovigilance Practices (GVP) modules). GVP modules replace Volume 9A, the previous EC guidance.

The roles and responsibilities of a MAH with regards to Pharmacovigilance include:

• To operate a pharmacovigilance system with documented procedures.
• Assure responsibility and liability for marketed products.
• To appoint a Qualified Person for Pharmacovigilance (QPPV) and ensure the QPPV is adequately supported.
• Adverse drug reaction (ADR) reporting and periodic safety update reporting (PSUR).

- To immediately inform regulatory authorities of any information which may change the risk benefit balance.
- To respond to requests for information from regulatory authorities.
- To manage and minimize risks with their medicines.

Penalties for failing to carry out the requirements of the legislation can result in a number of outcomes, which include inspection, formal warning, public naming, urgent safety restriction, suspension, fines, or criminal liability. General compliance with the principles of pharmacovigilance is monitored by regulatory authorities through inspections. There is a risk-based approach to inspections (either routine or triggered), and pharmacovigilance inspections can be conducted as part of a national inspection programme or as a request by the CHMP. The inspecting authority is normally from the country where the QPPV resides and inspection findings are described as:

- Critical: a deficiency in pharmacovigilance systems, practices or processes that adversely affects the rights, safety, or well-being of patients or that poses a potential serious risk to public health or that represents a serious violation of the applicable legislation and guidelines.
- Major: a deficiency that could potentially adversely affect or that could potentially pose a risk to public health or that represents a violation of applicable legislation and guidelines.
- Other: a deficiency that would not be expected to adversely affect the rights, safety, or well-being of patients.

Further reading

Medicines and Healthcare products Regulatory Agency (2009). *Good Pharmacovigilance Practice Guide*. Pharmaceutical Press.
⚥ http://ec.europa.eu/health/documents/eudralex/vol-9/index_en.htm
⚥ http://ec.europa.eu/health/human-use/pharmacovigilance/index_en.htm

Overview of reporting of adverse drug reactions

Why is adverse drug reaction reporting important?

Post-authorization reporting of suspected ADRs plays a critical role in detecting previously unrecognized side effects. ADR reports serve as an early warning system and guide further research to provide more robust evidence of causality and frequency.

What is included in an adverse drug reaction report?

ADR reports must contain four minimum elements to be considered valid for entry onto regulatory databases:
- A 'suspect' drug.
- A suspected reaction.
- Patient details (at least one of sex, age, weight, initials, or local identification number).
- An identifiable reporter.

In order to assist assessment, ADR reports should contain as much detail as possible regarding the medicines involved, the reaction(s), and relevant medical history.

Who reports, and how?

MAHs are required to submit reports to regulatory authorities electronically, using standards defined in ICH E2B. Healthcare professionals and patients are encouraged to report ADRs directly to national competent authorities (NCAs). Legal requirements for healthcare professionals vary within the EU.

European Union regulatory requirements for adverse drug reaction reporting

The requirements for post-authorization ADR reporting are defined in pharmacovigilance legislation. It is important to note that some details have recently changed after the implementation of new legislation in 2012 (note also that reporting requirements for the US FDA and Japanese MHLW are not identical to EU requirements). In particular, the definition of an ADR has been broadened to include those arising from medical error, off label use, drug abuse and drug misuse. MAHs must have adequate systems and trained personnel to ensure that ADR reports are collated, coded (using the MedDRA dictionary), and reconciled. MAH reporting requirements are set out in the relevant GVP modules. MAHs will report all ADRs to the Eudravigilance (EudraV) database.

National adverse drug reaction reporting schemes, e.g. UK Yellow Card Scheme

The UK MHRA operates the Yellow Card Scheme, placing particular emphasis on newly-authorized medicines. New EU-wide legislation implemented in 2012 is also set to focus additional monitoring on new drugs.

Serious adverse drug reactions

A 'serious' ADR is one that results in death, is life-threatening, requires or prolongs hospitalization, results in persistent or significant disability or incapacity, or is a congenital anomaly/birth defect:

- MAHs must submit serious ADR reports occurring within the EU to the relevant authorities within 15 days of initial receipt.
- NCAs must also submit the reports electronically to the Eudravigilance database within 15 days.
- MAHs must submit serious unexpected ADRs from non-EU countries within 15 days (unexpected = not already listed in the relevant EU Summary of Product Characteristics).

Follow-up of reports

Serious reports (including pregnancy exposures) should be followed-up for missing information, and additional data should be submitted according to a 15-day deadline.

- *Lack of efficacy* reports need not normally be expedited within 15 days, but this may be appropriate if efficacy is critical (e.g. for life-threatening diseases or vaccines).

Reports from studies

For post-authorization studies that qualify as clinical trials, the reporting criteria laid down in Clinical Trials Directive 2001/20/EC should be followed, in addition to PSUR requirements. For non-interventional studies the usual pharmacovigilance reporting criteria apply.

Non-prescription drugs

The Human Medicines Regulations 2012

The Human Medicines Regulations classifies medicines into three groups—prescription-only (POM) medicines, pharmacy medicines, and medicines classified as being on the general sales list (GSL). Both pharmacy medicines and GSL medicines may be sold without a prescription.

Pharmacy medicines

Pharmacy medicines can only be sold on site in a registered pharmacy, and their sale must be supervised by a registered pharmacist. They are only allowed to sell the medicine if the patient fits the criteria for it to be dispensed. The list of pharmacy medicines has increased greatly over the past few years and now includes the PDE-5 inhibitor, sildenafil, the proton pump inhibitor (PPI), omeprazole, emergency contraception, and other agents, such as tamsulosin, for treatment of benign prostatic hypertrophy (BPH) symptoms.

Rules are set to limit access to medicines where there may be an undiagnosed chronic illness. Examples include limits set around the numbers of purchases of thrush treatments, in case there is underlying diabetes mellitus, and recurrent purchases of indigestion therapies.

General sales list

Medicines on the general sales list may be sold in a wide range of shops including garages, newsagents, and supermarkets. Only small pack sizes or low strengths of medicines are admitted to the GSL, examples being paracetamol and ibuprofen, where pack sizes are 16 vs. 32 in the pharmacy for paracetamol, and maximum strength ibuprofen sold is 200 mg on the GSL, vs. 400 mg in the pharmacy medicine setting.

Lifecycle management

Lifecycle management, with switching of appropriate medicines from the prescription-only to the pharmacy list or from the pharmacy list to the GSL, is an important consideration, managing both the revenue stream from agents reaching the end of their patent life, and maximizing appropriate access for patients.

Proprietary Association of Great Britain

The Proprietary Association of Great Britain (PAGB) deals with the self-regulation of organizations producing OTC medicines. They have operated a pre-publication approval system for advertising materials for OTC medicines for the last 90 years. It is a condition of membership of the trade association that members submit their advertising for pre-approval.

The organization also regulates promotional materials for both food supplements and herbal medicines.

Further reading

📖 http://www.pagb.co.uk/codes/advertising.html

Chapter 2.28

Provision of unlicensed medicines

Overview

Legislation under European Law, which has been enacted in the UK under the Human Medicines Regulations, governs the provision of unlicenced medicines. An unlicenced medicine is one that is not licensed in the UK for human use in any indication or age group. Off-licence use of a medication involves use under a different indication or in a different population to that for which the medicine was originally licensed.

Duties of the pharmaceutical industry

Under the Human Medicines Regulations in the UK, and a similar legal framework across Europe and the US, industry has a legal obligation not to promote unlicenced medications or off-licence use of existing agents. The marketing authorization specifically states the indication for a particular medicine, and offers some protection to healthcare professionals who use it within the terms of the MA. Clause 3 of the Prescription Medicines Code of Practice Authority (PMCPA) Code of Practice deals with this with respect to self-regulation by industry.

Off-licence use of a medication

Medicines legislation does allow for use of a medicine in an off-licence setting by a registered medical practitioner. Essentially, it relies on the judgement of the physician with respect to benefit risk. The commonest situation where off-licence prescribing exists is in the paediatric population. Most agents were not studied historically in children; hence, clinicians themselves were responsible for developing modified dosing schedules for these medicines.

Compassionate-use programmes

Compassionate-use programmes are intended to allow patients access to potentially effective new medicines under development where options available in the EU are currently limited with respect to current therapies, and the disease being treated is chronic, serious, debilitating, or life-threatening. Specific guidance from EMA exists on these programmes.

The programmes are intended for groups of patients, rather than individuals, and the medicine concerned must be the subject of an application for marketing authorization under the centralized procedure, or be in late stage clinical trials in the EU.

Guidance from EMA states that such programmes should not hinder or slow down recruitment to clinical trial programmes, as whilst safety data can be collected from compassionate-use programmes, it cannot replace/substitute data from a clinical trial.

Named patient prescribing

Prescribing of a medication on a named-patient basis is slightly different from compassionate use. A decision to prescribe on a named-patient basis is taken by the prescriber on the basis that there is no licensed alternative for the particular condition/patients circumstances. The medication may have been previously available in the country concerned, but is no longer produced; it may be a specific formulation for the patient; supply problems may dictate that a licensed alternative is not available; or it may be for an orphan condition where a specific MA has not been applied for in the country where the patient resides, but one exists elsewhere.

Further reading

℘ http://www.pmcpa.org.uk/thecode/Pages/default.aspx
℘ http://www.emea.europa.eu/pdfs/human/euleg/2717006enfin.pdf
℘ http://www.emea.europa.eu/pdfs/human/pmf/2001–83-EC.pdf. Article 5 applies to named patient medicines.

Reclassification of medicines

Overview

The Human Medicines Regulations 2012 and Council Directive 2001/83/EC control the sale and supply of medicines. The legal status of medicinal products is part of the marketing authorization (MA) and products may be available either:

- On a prescription (POMs).
- Available in a pharmacy without prescription, under the supervision of a pharmacist (P).
- On General Sales List (GSL).

A new medicine, when first authorized, is usually restricted to use under medical supervision and made available only on a prescription (POM). If experience demonstrates that the medicine is safe for use with pharmacist supervision, reclassification as a P may be undertaken. If further experience demonstrates that access to professional advice is not required for safe use of the medicine, they may then be reclassified as GSL medicines to allow sale from a wider range of retail outlets.

The presumption under law is that all medicines are P unless they meet the criteria for POM or GSL status.

Switching from prescription-only to pharmacy medicines

Before a medicine can be switched from POM to P, ministers must be satisfied that it would be safe to allow it to be supplied without a prescription. In order for this to be possible, a medicine must no longer fulfill the following criteria:

- Be likely to present a direct or indirect danger to human health, even when used correctly, if used without the supervision of a doctor.
- Be frequently and to a very wide extent used incorrectly, and as a result is likely to present a direct or indirect danger to human health.
- Contain substances or preparations of substances of which the activity requires, or the side effects require, further investigation.
- Normally be prescribed by a doctor for parenteral administration (i.e. by injection).

The content of the reclassification application for POM to P should consist of the following elements:

- Reclassification application form.
- Reclassification summary: a comprehensive summary in set format, that will form part of the information, provided for the public consultation (Box 2.29.1).
- Safety/efficacy summary: supporting safety and where necessary efficacy data.
- Patient information: full details of leaflets and labels and an indication of the advertising plans.
- Training and education: a summary of what provision has been made for appropriate education and training.
- Clinical expert report: a critical evaluation of the proposed pharmacy product demonstrating that none of the prescription criteria apply.

> **Box 2.29.1 Reclassification summary for POM to P applications**
>
> 1. Applicant details.
> 2. Product details.
> 3. Rationale for the reclassification.
> 4. Support for reclassification.
> 5. Specific OTC requirements.
> 6. Safety profile.

Switching from pharmacy medicines (P) to general sales list (GSL)

Before a medicine can be switched from P to GSL, Ministers must be satisfied that it 'can with reasonable safety be sold or supplied otherwise than by or under the supervision of a pharmacist'.

The following classes of products are excluded from GSL:
- Anthelmintics.
- Parenterals.
- Eye drops.
- Eye ointments.
- Enemas.
- Irrigations used wholly or mainly for wounds, bladder, vagina, or rectum.
- Aspirin or aloxiprin for administration wholly or mainly to children.

The content of the reclassification application should consist of the following elements:
- Reclassification application form.
- Reclassification summary: a comprehensive summary in set format, which will form part of the information, provided for the public consultation (Box 2.29.2).
- Safety/efficacy summary: supporting safety and, where necessary, efficacy data.
- Patient information: full details of leaflets and labels, and an indication of the advertising plans.
- Clinical expert report: a critical evaluation of the proposed GSL product demonstrating that reclassification is both safe and necessary.

Box 2.29.2 Reclassification summary for P to GSL applications

1. Applicant details.
2. Product details.
3. Rationale for the reclassification.
4. Support for reclassification.
5. Specific GSL requirements.

Further reading

Directive 2001/83/EC of the European Parliament and of the Council of 6 November 2001 on the community code relating to medicinal products for human use. *Official Journal L*, **311**, 67–128.

MHRA Guidance Note 11: Changing the legal classification in the United Kingdom of a medicine for human use. Available at: ℘ http://www.mhra.gov.uk/Howweregulate/Medicines/Licensingofmedicines/Legalstatusandreclassification/index.htm

Parallel imports

Parallel importation

Parallel importation is a cross-border trade where importers supply products from lower-priced markets to customers in higher-priced markets, without the authorization of the intellectual property right holder. The products are not counterfeit or pirated. The parallel trade in pharmaceuticals has grown throughout the UK and other EU countries, and exists wherever there are significant price differentials between countries. Parallel importing is lawful in the EU, based on the principles of free movement of goods (Article 28 TFEU) and subject to the applicable derogations in EU law (Article 36 TFEU).

Medicinal products and devices

Parallel imported medicinal products must fulfil the necessary requirements of regulatory agencies. In the UK, the Parallel Import Licensing scheme allows medicinal products authorized in other member states to be marketed in the UK. However, the imported products must have no therapeutic difference from equivalent UK products.

The MHRA liaises with the other competent authorities to ensure that only products that conform to specific criteria are granted a licence. The imported medicinal product must be repackaged with an English language label and package leaflet (PL). In the UK, applications for parallel importation of medicinal products are divided into three categories:

- Simple: UK product and the imported product are manufactured by companies in the same group or are made under licence from the same licence holder.
- Standard: UK and imported products do not share a common origin.
- Complex: UK and imported products do not share a common origin and the imported product fulfils one or more other specific criteria. For example, the product to be imported contains a new excipient or sterilization method.

The processes for approving products for parallel trade are different for centrally authorized (EMA) products. Parallel trade of products licenced under the CP is referred to as parallel distribution.

Appropriately CE marked medical devices (EU conformity) can be marketed anywhere in the Community, provided that all the necessary requirements of the relevant Directive are fulfilled. Individual member states can prevent the free movement of a medical device if there is a particular safety or efficacy concern or if the pertinent regulatory requirements are not adhered to.

Further reading

℘ http://www.mhra.gov.uk/Howweregulate/Medicines/Licensingofmedicines/Parallelimportlicences/index.htm

℘ http://www.ema.europa.eu/htms/human/parallel/parallel.htm. Commission Communication on Parallel Imports: COM (2003) 839

Clinical pharmacology

Absorption, distribution, metabolism, and excretion

Overview

ADME stands for absorption, distribution, metabolism, and excretion, the 4 key processes that underlie pharmacokinetics. Pathophysiological disorders that affect any stage of this process, and characteristics of a medicine that affect any or multiple stages of this process can impact on the time concentration curve of the medicine and, thus, efficacy and toxicity.

Examples of the impact of the components of ADME and how they may impact on the development process are described below.

Absorption

For oral drugs, absorption is the extent to which a drug is absorbed from the gut lumen into the portal circulation. Two important features are the rate and extent of absorption. Examples of factors governing drug absorption from the gastrointestinal (GI) tract are shown in Table 3.1.1.

Table 3.1.1 Examples of factors governing drug absorption from the GI tract

Better absorption	Worse absorption
Low molecular weight	High molecular weight
Polar (acidic or basic)	Neutral

Examples of methods of delivery are shown in Table 3.1.2.

Table 3.1.2 Methods of delivery

Route	Example substance
Oral	Digoxin—low molecular weight, polar substance, well absorbed
Oral	Bisphosphonates—very high molecular weight, very poorly absorbed, low bioavailability
Transdermal	Testosterone patch—sustained delivery allows for gradual release of testosterone, preferable to injections
Pulmonary	Insulin—subject to degradation by stomach enzymes, insulin efficiently absorbed by respiratory mucosa

Distribution

Distribution refers to the process of the drug moving into and out of the tissues of the body. The volume of distribution relates the concentration of the drug in the plasma to the total amount of the drug in the body. Examples of factors that may impact on volume of distribution are shown in Table 3.1.3.

Table 3.1.3 Factors that may impact on volume of distribution (examples)

Low volume of distribution	Large volume of distribution
Highly protein bound	Low protein binding
Low level of lipophilicity	Highly lipophilic (increased tissue binding)

Metabolism

Metabolism describes the processes (biotransformation) that change the drug into another molecule. In general these processes can be classified as Phase I and Phase II reactions. The liver is the principal organ of drug metabolism. Many examples exist that impact as CYP-450 enzyme inhibitors or inducers, leading to reduced or increased drug concentrations. Four examples are detailed in Table 3.1.4. A fuller list of the main CYP-450 inhibitors/inducers can be found at the online version of the P450 Drug Interaction Table.

Table 3.1.4 Examples of CYP-450 enzyme inhibitors or inducers

Drug/class	Inhibitor/inducer
Macrolide—erythromycin, clarithromycin	CYP-450 3A4 inhibitors
Fruit juices (cranberry/grapefruit)	Inhibitors of CYP-2C8 / CYP 3A4
Herbal antidepressant (St John's Wort)	CYP-450 enzyme inducer
Carbamazepine	CYP-450 enzyme inducer

Excretion

Excretion describes the processes that remove the drug from the body. A number of routes for drug excretion exist. Examples are given in Table 3.1.5.

Table 3.1.5 Example routes for drug excretion

Route	Example
Hepatic	Pancuronium
Pulmonary	Enfluorane
Renal—Passive filtration	Digoxin
Renal—anionic active transporter	Oseltamivir
Renal—cationic active transporter	Famotidine
Renal transport inhibitor	Dapafloglozin—SGLT-2 inhibitor

Each aspect of pharmacokinetic (PK) is important in clinical development and we explore each aspect of ADME in pre-clinical and clinical development.

Further reading

🔊 http://medicine.iupui.edu/clinpharm/ddis/table.aspx

Volume of distribution, clearance, half-life

Volume of distribution

The apparent volume of distribution (Vd) is the theoretical volume of fluid into which the total drug administered would have to be diluted to produce the concentration in plasma. Volume of distribution has nothing to do with the actual volume of the body or its fluid compartments but rather involves the distribution of the drug within the body (see example in Box 3.2.1).

Box 3.2.1 Example

If 500 mg of a drug is given and the plasma concentration measures 10 mg/L, 500 mg seems to be distributed in 50 L (dose/volume = concentration; 500 mg/$\times$ L = 10 mg/L).

Volume of distribution provides little information about the pattern of distribution of a drug. However, if a drug remains in the circulation, it will have a low Vd. For drugs that are highly tissue-bound, comparatively little of a dose remains in the circulation to be measured; thus, plasma concentration is low and volume of distribution is high. Each drug is uniquely distributed in the body.

Many acidic drugs (e.g. warfarin) are highly protein-bound and stay in the plasma, and thus have a small apparent volume of distribution. Many basic drugs (e.g. amphetamine) are extensively taken up by tissues and, thus, have an apparent volume of distribution larger than the volume of the entire body.

Clearance

Drug clearance (CL) is defined as the volume of plasma in the vascular compartment cleared of drug per unit time by the processes of metabolism and excretion. Clearance, therefore, the measure of the ability of the body to eliminate a drug. Clearance is expressed as a volume per unit of time. It is usually further defined as blood clearance (CL_b), plasma clearance (CL_p), or clearance based on the concentration of unbound or free drug (CL_u), depending on the concentration measured.

Clearance by means of various organs of elimination is additive. Elimination of drug may occur as a result of processes that occur in the liver, kidney, and other organs. Added together, these separate clearances will equal total systemic clearance:

$$Cl_{hepatic} + CL_{renal} + CL_{other} = CL_{total}$$

Other routes of elimination could include that in saliva or sweat, partition into the gut, and metabolism at sites other than the liver (e.g., nitroglycerin, which is metabolized in all tissues of the body).

Half-life

The half-life ($t_{1/2}$) is the time it takes for the plasma concentration or the amount of drug in the body to be reduced by 50% and is determined by both the volume of distribution and clearance. Experimentally, the half-life can be determined by giving a single dose, usually IV, and then the concentration of the drug in the plasma is measured at regular intervals. The concentration of the drug will reach a peak value in the plasma (Cmax) and will then fall as the drug is broken down and cleared from the blood (see Fig. 3.2.1).

The time taken for the plasma concentration to halve is the half-life of that drug. Some drugs like ibuprofen have very short half-lives, others, like warfarin and digoxin, take much longer to eliminate from the plasma, resulting in a long half-life. So drugs like ibuprofen that are cleared from the blood more rapidly than others need to be given in regular doses to build up and maintain a high enough concentration in the blood to be therapeutically effective.

As repeated doses of a drug are administered, its plasma concentration builds up and reaches what is known as a steady state (see Fig. 3.2.2). This is when the amount of drug in the plasma has built up to a concentration level that is therapeutically effective and as long as regular doses are administered to balance the amount of drug being cleared the drug will continue to be active. The time taken to reach the steady state is about five times the half-life of a drug. Drugs like digoxin and warfarin with a long half-life will take longer to reach a steady state than drugs with a shorter half-life.

Sometimes a loading dose may be administered so that a steady state is reached more quickly. Then smaller 'maintenance' doses are given to ensure that the drug levels stay within the steady state.

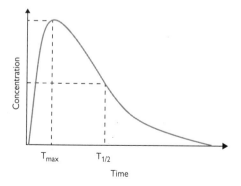

Fig. 3.2.1 Concentration of a drug in blood plasma over time.

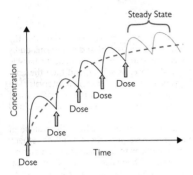

Fig. 3.2.2 The steady state.

Further reading

Beers MH, Porter RS, Jones TV, Kaplan JL, Berkwits M, eds. (2006). *The Merck Manual of Diagnosis and Therapy.* 18th edn. NJ: Whitehouse Station: Merck Research Laboratories; 2006.

Pre-clinical aspects of pharmacokinetics

Absorption

Several models are in development/validation for pre-clinical study of intestinal drug absorption. Those under validation include *in situ* perfusion models utilizing small intestine from rodents and other mammalian species.

Distribution

Computational models exist that can extrapolate data from small animal studies to a comparable human situation. In general, distribution data is obtained from whole animal studies.

Metabolism

Various models exist with respect to evaluation of liver metabolism. These include liver microsomes, cultured whole cell liver preparations, and perfused liver slices where liver architecture is preserved. These allow study of both phase I and phase II liver metabolism, including cytochrome P450 induction/inhibition.

Excretion

The major concern with respect to excretion is interaction with renal organic anion transporters (OATs) and cation transporters. Knockout animal models now exist for each of the OATs. As yet, 7 or more OATs have been identified, with varying tissue expression, including the kidney.

How many species should pharmacokinetics data be demonstrated in?

Regulatory guidance suggests that PK data should be demonstrated in two species prior to the first time in human studies. It is most usual to conduct studies in the rat and the dog with respect to small molecule development. With respect to biologicals, species applicability will almost certainly dictate the need for PK data in a monkey model prior to moving into first time in human studies.

What are the key pieces of pharmacokinetics data required?

- Cmax: peak serum concentration reached.
- Tmax: time to reach peak drug concentration.
- AUC: area under the concentration time curve: measure of total drug exposure.
- Half-life: time taken for serum concentration to reduce by 50% from peak.
- Oral bioavailability: central compartment drug concentration adminstered orally, as a percentage of the same dose administered IV.
- Volume of distribution: theoretical volume of fluid into which the total drug administered would have to be diluted to produce the measured plasma concentration.
- Steady state concentration: plasma drug concentration reached after a number of administrations.

Chapter 3.4

Non-clinical data

Non-clinical data

Non-clinical data is research data generated from in vitro laboratory studies and from in vivo studies in animals. The data help characterize the important pharmacokinetic (what the body does to the drug) and pharmacodynamic (what the drug does to the body) features of a medicinal product. Non-clinical data is also used to help predict the expected toxicity profile and this is of paramount importance for first-in-man studies. In such cases, assessment of non-clinical data influences the decision to proceed with a clinical trial.

Clinical data often supersedes non-clinical data during the later stages of the development programme of a new medicinal product. However, some characteristics of a medicinal product cannot be ethically researched in humans (reproductive toxicity, carcinogenic potential, and genotoxicity). For regulatory submissions, a detailed non-clinical overview must be included in Module 2 of the dossier. The overview will include reference to GLP compliance and detailed description of the experimental systems, results, and overall conclusions.

Points to consider in the assessment of non-clinical data

- Statutory requirements such as ICH guidelines, scientific advice/ protocol assistance and GLP compliance.
- Physical chemistry of the medicinal product.
- Pharmacokinetics:
  - methods of analysis and validation;
  - absorption—site of absorption, single/repeat dose kinetics, dose proportionality, absolute bioavailability;
  - distribution—tissue and blood cell distribution, protein binding, distribution in relation to possible target organs;
  - metabolism—structures and quantities of metabolites, metabolic pathways, in vitro metabolism;
  - excretion—routes of excretion, organ specific toxicity, mass balance;
  - PK drug interactions—focus on drugs that are potentially going to be co-administered in man.
- Primary and secondary pharmacodynamics: proof of concept and mode of action, therapeutic activity, duration/reversibility of effects, activity of metabolites, immunological properties, receptor screens.
- Safety pharmacology: the relevance of the animal species for human safety assessment, predicting potential adverse events in humans.
- Toxicity:
  - single dose toxicity studies—duration of observation, clinical signs of acute toxicity, the approximate lethal dose or observed maximum non-lethal dose;
  - repeat dose toxicity studies—exposure margin (comparability of observed systemic exposure in the animal model to the proposed systemic exposure in man);

- • genotoxicity—mutagenicity, chromosomal aberrations, primary DNA damage, exposure, in vitro and in vivo testing;
  - • carcinogenicity—lifespan studies, neoplastic, and non-neoplastic changes, statistical analysis of data.
- Reproductive and developmental toxicity: margins of exposure and the clinical relevance of the findings, fertility and early embryonic development, embryo-fetal development, pre- and post-natal development (including maternal function), offspring (juvenile animals).
- Local tolerance: evidence of local irritancy at the site of administration.
- Other studies as appropriate:
  - antigenicity;
  - immunotoxicity;
  - dependency;
  - metabolites and impurities;
  - phototoxicity.
- Environmental risk assessment (ERA): potential risks to the environment, recommendations for mitigation measures

Further reading

Cartwright, Anthony C., Matthews, Brian R (2009). *International Pharmaceutical Product Registration*, 2nd edn. London: Informa Healthcare.
 http://www.ich.org/

Clinical aspects of pharmacokinetics

Overview

The direction of clinical studies to generate PK data depends upon evaluation of the pre-clinical data package. Key aspects to be considered include:

- Pharmacological basis of principal effects (mechanism of action).
- Dose–response or concentration–response relationships and duration of action.
- Study of the potential clinical routes of administration.
- Systemic general pharmacology, including pharmacological effects on major organ systems and physiological responses.
- Studies of ADME in pre-clinical models.

The place of pharmacokinetic studies in the development programme

EMA regulatory guidelines: Phase I

PK may be assessed via separate studies or as a part of efficacy, safety, and tolerance studies. PK studies are particularly important to assess the clearance of the drug and to anticipate possible accumulation of parent drug or metabolites, and potential drug–drug interactions.

Studies conducted in later phases of development

- Food effect on bioavailability.
- Subpopulation PK, e.g. in renal/hepatic impairment.
- Drug–drug interaction studies.

Special considerations

Studies of drug metabolites

Major active metabolite(s) should be identified and deserve detailed PK study. Timing of the metabolite assessment studies within the development plan depends on the characteristics of the individual drug.

Drug–drug interaction

If a potential for drug–drug interaction is suggested by metabolic profile, studies on drug interaction during clinical development are highly recommended. For drugs that are frequently co-administered, it is usually important that drug–drug interaction studies be performed in non-clinical and, if appropriate in human studies. This is particularly true for drugs that are known to alter the absorption or metabolism of other drugs (see ICH E7), or whose metabolism or excretion can be altered by effects by other drugs.

Special populations

In addition to studies in patients with hepatic or renal impairment, studies in ethnic subgroups, and the in the elderly population are recommended.

Further reading

European Medicines Agency (1998). General considerations for clinical trials. Available at: ℜ http://www.ema.europa.eu/docs/en_GB/document_library/Scientific_guideline/2009/09/ WC500002877.pdf (ICH E8)

Dose–response relationship

Overview

The dose–response relationship is the measurement of the relationship between the dose of a substance administered and its overall effect (the response), either therapeutic or toxic. The dose–response relationship is based on observed data from experimental animal, human clinical, or cell studies. Generally, the higher the dose, the greater the response.

Knowledge of the dose–response relationship is important as it helps:

- Establish causality that the drug has, in fact, induced the observed effects.
- Establish the lowest dose where an induced effect occurs—the threshold effect.
- Determines the rate at which response/toxic effect builds up—the slope for the dose response.

Dose–response curve

The dose–response curve normally takes the form of a sigmoid curve as shown in Fig. 3.6.1.

The point at which a response first appears is known as the threshold dose level. An important aspect of dose–response relationships is the concept of threshold. Using dose response curves, one can examine the threshold for both effective dose (ED) and toxic dose (TD) in determining the relative safety of pharmaceuticals. As shown below, two dose–response curves are presented for the same drug, one for effectiveness and the other for toxicity. In this case, a dose that is 50% effective (ED50) does not cause toxicity whereas a 90% effective dose (ED90) may result in a significant amount of toxicity.

As can be seen in Fig. 3.6.2, there is a dose below which there are no adverse effects from exposure to the drug. This is called the no observed adverse effect level (NOAEL). A NOAEL is the highest exposure level at which no statistically or biologically significant increases are seen in the frequency or severity of adverse effect between the exposed population and its appropriate control population. In cases in which a NOAEL has not

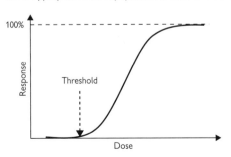

Fig. 3.6.1 The dose–response curve.

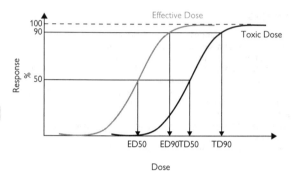

Fig. 3.6.2 The no observed adverse effect level (NOAEL).

been demonstrated experimentally, the term 'lowest observed adverse effect level (LOAEL)' is used, which is the lowest dose tested.

Therapeutic index

The concept of therapeutic index refers to the relationship between toxic and therapeutic dose.

The therapeutic index of a drug is the ratio of the dose that produces toxicity to the dose that produces a clinically desired or effective response in a population of individuals (see Fig. 3.6.3). A higher therapeutic index is preferable to a lower one: a patient would have to take a much higher dose of such a drug to reach the lethal/toxic threshold than the dose taken to elicit the therapeutic effect.

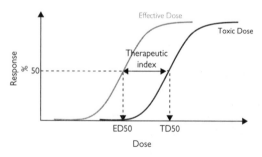

Fig. 3.6.3 The Therapeutic index.

Generally, a drug or other therapeutic agent with a narrow therapeutic range (i.e. having little difference between toxic and therapeutic doses) may have its dosage adjusted according to measurements of the actual blood levels achieved in the person taking it. This may be achieved through therapeutic drug monitoring (TDM) protocols. Some drugs with a narrow therapeutic index are shown in Box 3.6.1.

Box 3.6.1 Some drugs with a narrow therapeutic index

- Warfarin.
- Lithium.
- Digoxin.
- Phenytoin.
- Gentamycin.
- Amphotericin B.
- 5-fluorouracil.
- AZT.

Proof of concept studies

Overview

A proof of concept study is designed to deliver evidence of efficacy in a small number of selected patients. It is designed to provide the confidence to progress to later studies, with the minimal possible investment, and with results delivered in the shortest possible time.

Objectives for a proof of concept study:

- Validation of a novel therapeutic target and in vivo pre-clinical models to the target population.
- Identification of potential surrogates for efficacy or toxicity.
- Provide early evidence of clinical efficacy.
- Earlier elimination of a non-viable target from the pipeline.
- Guide potential target populations and hence potential commercial return.

Prospective setting of Go/No-go criteria is crucial, areas where criteria that may impact include:

- Safety.
- Tolerability.
- Pharmacokinetics.
- Duration of action.
- Dose/pharmacodynamics (PD) relationship.
- Clinical efficacy.
- Patient acceptability.
- Commercial viability in the indication at potential time of launch.

Bayesian statistics

Bayesian statistics play an increasingly important role in proof of concept study design, allowing the determination of conditional probability. They allow for interim analysis and removal of ineffective dose regimens or, indeed, early termination of a study if futility is suggested.

Study size and duration

Study size and duration depends on the disease indication and the potential biological effect size, and the degree of risk the organization is prepared to take with respect to moving on to further studies. For many studies, a pre-determined point estimate deemed as success is set and confidence intervals for success are set where $\frac{2}{3}$ to $\frac{3}{4}$ of the treated population is predicted to lie above the no significant effect line.

Further reading

Smith MK, Jones I, Morris MF, Grieve AP, Tan K (2006). Implementation of a Bayesian adaptive design in a proof of concept study, *Pharmaceutical Statistics* **5**(1) 39–50. Available at: http://onlinelibrary.wiley.com/doi/10.1002/pst.198/abstract

Reproductive toxicity studies

Overview

The aim of studies is to reveal any effect of a new active substance on mammalian reproduction. Data should be used in association with other toxicological data in risk assessment.

Studies should evaluate exposure to mature adults and at all stages of development (see Table 3.8.1).

- Pre-mating to conception (fertility/early embryonic development [FEED]).
- Conception to implantation (FEED).
- Implantation to closure of hard palate (embryo-fetal toxicity [EFT]).
- Closure of hard palate to end of pregnancy (pre- and postnatal development [PPN]).
- Birth to weaning (PPN).
- Weaning to sexual maturity (PPN).

Fertility/early embryonic development

These studies test for toxic effects from treatment before mating, through mating to implantation. These tests are performed in one species, usually rat. Animals are dosed for 2 weeks before mating (females) or 4 weeks (males) through post-mating (males) or implantation (females)

Females are sacrificed at days 13–15 to allow assessment of implantation/resorption. Males are sacrificed once the outcome of mating has been confirmed.

Observations carried out include:

- Macroscopic and microscopic examination of reproductive organs.
- Sperm count/viability.
- Implantation sites/corpora lutea.
- Number of viable fetuses.

FEED data is required in males before phase III in all region. In females, data is required before phase III in US and EU, and before any inclusion in women of child-bearing potential (WOCBP) in any trial in Japan.

Embryo-fetal toxicity

Pregnant females dosed from implantation to closure of hard palate to assess effect on pregnant female and embryo-fetal development. Performed in 2 species, one rodent (usually rat) and one non-rodent (usually rabbit).

Three dose levels are usually assessed and preliminary pharmacokinetic evaluation undertaken. Females are sacrificed one day before parturition and fetuses examined for abnormalities.

In the EU, these studies are required before WOCBP are allowed into clinical trials. In the USA, WOCBP with adequate contraception are allowed into trials without this data up to, but not including, phase III.

Table 3.8.1 Reproductive toxicity studies by phase of development

Stage of development	Studies required	Species required	Phase required	Observations
Premating to conception	FEED	1	• Males before phase III	• Macro/microscopic examination of reproductive organs
Conception to implantation		Usually rat	• Females before phase III in US and EU, before any inclusion in WOCBP in any trial in Japan	• Sperm count/viability • Implantation sites/corpora lutea • No of viable fetuses
Implantation to closure of hard palate	EFT	2 One rodent (usually rat) One non-rodent (usually rabbit)	• EU before WOCBP in trials • In US up to phase 3 with adequate contraception	• Fetuses examined for abnormalities
Closure of hard palate end of pregnancy Birth to weaning Weaning to sexual maturity	PPN	1 Usually rat	• Before submission for MAA or earlier if any concerns identified	Implantations, number of offspring, pre-post weaning survival/growth, physical development, sensory function/behaviour

Data from ICH S5(R2), Detection of toxicity to reproduction for medicinal products and toxicity to male fertility. Available at: ® http://www.ich.org/fileadmin/Public_Web_Site/ICH_Products/Guidelines/Safety/S5_R2/Step4/S5_R2_Guideline.pdf

Pre- and postnatal development

These test for adverse effects on:
• Pregnant lactating females.
• Fetuses/offspring until sexual maturity.

They are performed in one species (usually rat). Pregnant females are dosed from implantation to the end of lactation. Maternal animals are assessed for:
• Implantations.
• Number of offspring.
• Pre-post weaning survival/growth.
• Physical development.
• Sensory function and behaviour.

Studies should be completed before submission for MAA or earlier if any concerns identified.

Further reading

ICH Harmonised Tripartite Guidelines.
ICH S5(R2). Detection of toxicity to reproduction for medicinal products and toxicity to male fertility. Available at ℘ http: www.ich.org
ICH M3(R1). Guideline on non-clinical safety studies for the conduct of human clinical trials for pharmaceuticals. Available at ℘ http: www.ich.org

Immunotoxicity testing

Overview

ICH Topic S8: Guidance on immunotoxicity studies for human pharmaceuticals, states that evaluation of potential adverse effects of human pharmaceuticals on the immune system should be incorporated into standard drug development.

Toxicity to the immune system includes suppression or enhancement of the immune response. Suppression of the immune response can lead to decreased host resistance to infectious agents or tumour cells. Enhancing the immune response can exaggerate autoimmune diseases or hypersensitivity.

Immunosuppression or enhancement can be associated with two distinct groups:

- Drugs intended to modulate immune function for therapeutic purposes (e.g. to prevent organ transplant rejection) where adverse immunosuppression can be considered exaggerated pharmacodynamics.
- Drugs not intended to affect immune function, but cause immunotoxicity due, for example, to necrosis of immune cells.

Immunotoxicity studies

Factors to consider that might prompt additional immunotoxicity studies can be identified in the following areas (see Fig. 3.9.1).

- Findings from standard toxicity studies:
  - haematological changes;
  - alterations in immune system organ weights;
  - changes in serum globulins that occur without a plausible explanation;
  - increased incidence of infections;
  - increased occurrence of tumours.
- The pharmacological properties of the drug: if the pharmacological properties of a test compound indicate it has the potential to affect immune function (e.g. anti-inflammatory drugs), additional immunotoxicity testing should be considered.
- The intended patient population: additional immunotoxicity studies might be warranted if the majority of the patient population for whom the drug is intended is immunocompromised.
- Structural similarities to known immunomodulators.
- The disposition of the drug: if the compound and/or its metabolites are retained at high concentrations in cells of the immune system.
- Clinical information: clinical findings suggestive of immunotoxicity in patients exposed to the drug.

Standard toxicity studies

Table 3.9.1 lists the parameters that should be evaluated in standard toxicity studies for signs of immunotoxicity.

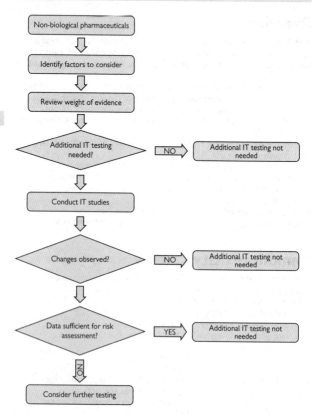

Fig. 3.9.1 Flow diagram for recommended immunotoxicity evaluation.

Additional immunotoxicity studies

T-cell dependent antibody response (TDAR)
The TDAR should be performed using a recognized T-cell dependent antigen (e.g. sheep red blood cells [SRBC]) or keyhole limpet haemocyanin [KLH]) that results in a robust antibody response.

Immunophenotyping
Immunophenotyping is the identification and/or enumeration of leukocyte subsets using antibodies. Immunophenotyping is usually conducted by flow cytometric analysis or by immunohistochemistry.

Table 3.9.1 Parameters for evaluation in standard toxicity studies

Parameter	Specific component
Haematology	Total and absolute differential leucocyte count
Clinical chemistry	Globulin level and A/G ratio
Gross pathology	Lymphoid organs/tissue
Organ weights	Thymus, spleen
Histology	Thymus, spleen, drainage, and one other lymph node, bone marrow, peyers patch, bronchus associated lymphoid tissue, nasal associated lymphoid tissue

Natural killer cell activity assays

Natural killer (NK) cell activity assays can be conducted if immunopheno-typing studies demonstrate a change in number, or if STS studies demonstrate increased viral infection rates, or in response to other factors.

Host resistance studies

Host resistance studies involve challenging groups of mice or rats treated with the different doses of test compound with varying concentrations of a pathogen (bacteria, fungal, viral, parasitic) or tumour cells. Models have been developed to evaluate a wide range of pathogens, such as *Listeria monocytogenes*, *Streptococcus pneumoniae*, *Candida albicans*, influenza virus, cytomegalovirus, *Plasmodium yoelii*, and *Trichinella spiralis*. Tumour host resistance models in mice have used the B16F10 melanoma and PYB6 sarcoma tumour cell lines.

Macrophage/neutrophil function

In vitro macrophage and neutrophil function assays (phagocytosis, oxidative burst, chemotaxis, and cytolytic activity) have been published for several species. These assays assess macrophage/neutrophil function of cells exposed to the test compound in vitro or obtained from animals treated with the test compound (ex vivo assay).

Assays to measure cell-mediated immunity

Assays to measure cell-mediated immunity have not been as well established as those used for the antibody response. These are in vivo assays where antigens are used for sensitization. The endpoint is the ability of drugs to modulate the response to challenge.

Further reading

ICH Topic S8. Immunotoxicity studies for human pharmaceuticals, note for guidance on immuno-toxicity studies for human pharmaceuticals CHMP/167235/2004. Available at ℘ www.ich.org

Chapter 3.10

Carcinogenicity

Carcinogenicity

Carcinogenicity is the ability or tendency to cause cancer. A carcinogen is a substance that is capable of increasing the incidence of a tumour or is able to shorten the time to tumour occurrence. The principal objective of carcinogenicity studies is to identify the carcinogenic potential of medicinal products, as part of the assessment of risk for an MAA (ICH Topics S1A, S1B, and S1C).

Carcinogenicity studies

Carcinogenicity studies should normally be performed for any medicinal product whose expected clinical use is continuous for at least 6 months or may be expected to be used repeatedly in an intermittent fashion. Studies should also be considered for products with a known class carcinogenic potential, where the structure activity relationship suggests a carcinogenic risk, if there is evidence of pre-neoplastic lesions in repeat dose toxicity studies or long-term tissue retention results in inflammatory responses. Genotoxicity studies provide a good indication of carcinogenic potential and unequivocally genotoxic compounds, in the absence of other data, are presumed to be carcinogens.

Medicinal products

Medicinal products administered infrequently or for short periods do not necessarily require carcinogenicity studies, and in instances where life-expectancy is short, long-term carcinogenicity studies may not be required. For medicinal products developed to treat certain serious diseases, carcinogenicity testing may not need to be conducted before market approval, but as a post-approval commitment. Carcinogenicity studies are not usually needed for endogenous substances given solely as replacement therapy and standard carcinogenicity studies are generally inappropriate for biotechnology-derived pharmaceuticals. However, product-specific assessment of carcinogenic potential may still be required if there is a biological concern.

Carcinogenicity studies

The basic scheme comprises one long-term rodent carcinogenicity study, plus one other supplementary study that provides additional information not readily available from the long-term study (e.g. transgenic mice predisposed to developing tumours). Emphasis is placed on the selection of a model that contributes the most important information to the overall weight of evidence for the assessment of carcinogenic potential. Whatever model is selected, it is imperative that an accurate knowledge of the background incidence of tumour is known.

Route of exposure

The route of exposure in animals should be the same as the intended clinical route and relevant target organs should be adequately exposed to the test product. Topically medicinal products may need carcinogenicity studies, although products showing poor systemic exposure may not need oral route studies. 50 animals of each sex are commonly used at three dose levels. Selected doses should allow an adequate margin of safety over human therapeutic exposure, be tolerated without significant chronic physiological dysfunction and permit data interpretation in the context of therapeutic use. Typically a double-sized concurrent control group is used.

Good laboratory practice

Frequent clinical observation and careful record keeping are essential. Autopsy and histopathological assessment should be carried out meticulously, with peer review of the slides. Both the incidence and time to tumour detection are compared between test and control groups, using pre-specified statistical analyses. Mechanistic studies are often useful for the interpretation of tumour findings and can provide a perspective on the relevance to human risk.

Further reading

℘ http://www.ich.org/products/guidelines/safety/article/safety-guidelines.html
℘ http://www.ema.europa.eu/pdfs/human/swp/287700en.pdf

Genotoxicity testing

Overview

Registration of pharmaceuticals requires a comprehensive assessment of their genotoxic potential. Genotoxicity tests can be defined as in vitro and in vivo tests designed to detect compounds that induce genetic damage by various mechanisms. These enable hazard identification with respect to fixation of damage to DNA in the form of:

- Gene mutations.
- Larger scale chromosomal damage.
- Recombination.

These are considered essential for heritable effects and in the multi-step process of malignancy. Numerical chromosome changes have also been associated with tumorigenesis and can indicate a potential for aneuploidy in germ cells.

Compounds that are positive in tests that detect such kinds of damage have the potential to be human carcinogens and/or mutagens. Because the relationship between exposure to particular chemicals and carcinogenesis is established for humans, genotoxicity tests have been used mainly for the prediction of carcinogenicity.

The standard test battery for genotoxicity

It is clear that no single test is capable of detecting all relevant genotoxic agents. Therefore, the usual approach should be to carry out a battery of in vitro and in vivo tests for genotoxicity. Such tests are complementary, rather than representing different levels of hierarchy. The following standard test battery is recommended based upon the considerations mentioned above:

- A test for gene mutation in bacteria.
- An in vitro test with cytogenetic evaluation of chromosomal damage with mammalian cells or an in vitro mouse lymphoma TK assay.
- An in vivo test for chromosomal damage using rodent haematopoietic cells.

A test for gene mutation in bacteria

It is appropriate to assess genotoxicity in a bacterial reverse mutation test. This test has been shown to detect relevant genetic changes and the majority of genotoxic rodent carcinogens.

An in vitro test with cytogenetic evaluation of chromosomal damage with mammalian cells or an in vitro mouse lymphoma TK assay

DNA damage considered to be relevant for mammalian cells and not adequately measured in bacteria should be evaluated in mammalian cells. Several mammalian cell systems are in use:

- Systems that detect gross chromosomal damage: in vitro tests for structural and numerical chromosomal aberrations.

- Systems that detect primarily gene mutation: test approaches currently accepted for the assessment of mammalian cell gene mutation involve the *tk* locus using mouse lymphoma L5178Y cells or human lymphoblastoid TK6 cells, the *hprt* locus using CHO cells, V79 cells, or L5178Y cells, or the *gpt* locus using AS52 cells.
- Systems that detects gene mutations and clastogenic effects: mouse lymphoma TK assay.

An in vivo test for chromosomal damage using rodent haematopoietic cells

Additional relevant factors (absorption, distribution, metabolism, excretion) that may influence the genotoxic activity of a compound are included. As a result, in vivo tests permit the detection of some additional genotoxic agents. An in vivo test for chromosomal damage in rodent haematopoietic cells fulfills this need.

This in vivo test for chromosomal damage in rodents could be either:

- Annalysis of chromosomal aberrations in bone marrow cells. *Or*
- Analysis of micronuclei in bone marrow or peripheral blood erythrocytes.

Modifications of the 3-test battery

There are situations where the standard 3-test battery may need modification.

Limitations to the use of bacterial test organisms

There are circumstances (e.g. compounds that are excessively toxic to bacteria) where the performance of the bacterial reverse mutation test does not provide appropriate or sufficient information for the assessment of genotoxicity. For these cases, usually two in vitro mammalian cell tests should be performed using two different cell types.

Compounds bearing structural alerts for genotoxic activity

Compounds bearing structural alerts that have given negative results in the standard 3-test battery may necessitate limited additional testing. The choice of additional test(s) or protocol modification(s) depends on the chemical nature, the known reactivity, and metabolism data on the structurally alerting compound under question.

Limitations to the use of standard in vivo tests

There are compounds for which standard in vivo tests do not provide additional useful information. These include compounds for which data from studies on toxicokinetics or pharmacokinetics indicate that they are not systemically absorbed and therefore are not available for the target tissues in standard in vivo genotoxicity tests. (For example, some dermally applied pharmaceuticals). In cases where a modification of the route of administration does not provide sufficient target tissue exposure, it may be appropriate to base the evaluation only on in vitro testing.

Additional genotoxicity testing in relation to the carcinogenicity

Bioassay

- *Evidence for tumour response:* additional genotoxicity testing in appropriate models may be conducted for compounds that were negative in the standard 3-test battery, but which have shown effects in carcinogenicity bioassay.
- *Structurally unique chemical classes:* on rare occasions, a completely novel compound in a unique structural chemical class will be introduced as a pharmaceutical. When such a compound will not be tested in chronic rodent carcinogenicity bioassays, further genotoxicity evaluation may be invoked.

Further reading

ICH Topic S2 (R1) (2012). Guidance on genotoxicity testing and data interpretation for pharmaceuticals intended for human use. Available at: ℜ http// www.ich.org.

Local tolerance

Local tolerance

Local tolerance studies aim to determine the potential effects of a medicinal product (active substance and excipients) at a site of application. In general, local tolerance studies should be designed to reflect the proposed clinical administration in man. In some circumstances, studies normally conducted on animals may be substituted by validated in vitro tests.

Local tolerance testing of medicinal products is rarely performed in isolation and the assessment is usually part of a battery of other toxicity studies (ICH M3). The testing method should be designed to distinguish physicochemical and mechanical effects of administration from toxicological and pharmacodynamic effects. The evaluation of local tolerance should, in most cases, be performed prior to human exposure.

Systemic toxicity testing

For novel products, evaluation of systemic toxicity will usually be conducted if the medicinal product has not been subject to previous toxicology investigation. The evaluation should utilize a route of administration that results in an appropriate level of systemic exposure. However, studies for the evaluation of systemic toxicity may not be required if:
- The absorption of the product is so low that the prospect of systemic effects can be discounted.
- The product is absorbed, but systemic toxicity has been previously demonstrated to a satisfactory level.

Site of administration

Tolerance testing should be established in areas that will come into contact with the medicinal product and in areas that may come into contact, either through unavoidable or accidental exposure. Sites of administration include:
- Oral.
- Dermal.
- Rectal.
- IV and intra-arterial.
- Ocular.
- Vaginal.
- Inhalation (intra-tracheal, intra-nasal, and pulmonary).
- Intra-vesicular.

Local tolerance tests

The choice of species will depend on the overall test model considered appropriate. The route of administration and the frequency and duration of administration should be selected according to the envisaged administration in man and the proposed clinical conditions of use. The product to be tested should be as similar as possible to the proposed clinical formulation. The dosing should include the concentration of the active substance to be used in man and the test should evaluate the degree of reversibility of any observed local lesions. Animal welfare is important and care should be taken to minimize painful exposure.

Further reading

ICH Safety Guidelines. Available at: ℘ http://www.ich.org/products/guidelines/safety/article/safety-guidelines.html

Committee for Proprietary Medicinal Products. Notes for guidance on non-clinical local tolerance testing of medicinal products. Available at: ℘ http://www.ema.europa.eu/pdfs/human/swp/214500en.pdf

Chapter 3.13

Acute toxicity

Overview

Acute toxicity testing involves the determination of adverse effects of an investigational agent within 24h of first administration. Traditionally acute toxicity has been assessed with single dose studies.

Most recently, however, EMA guidance has suggested that single dose toxicity studies should not now be conducted as they are of limited value, and obtaining data from the early period of multiple dosing studies is more acceptable with respect to animal welfare.

In most cases, acute toxicity can be assessed based on data from appropriately conducted dose–escalation studies or short-duration dose–ranging studies. You can therefore plan for collection of data on acute toxicity when designing dose–escalation or short-duration dose–ranging studies. Data from one species and following use of one route of administration are generally considered sufficient.

Subacute toxicity testing

Subacute toxicity testing involves the administration of multiple doses of an investigational agent.

At least 3 doses of agent are recommended, preferably 4 or 5 for both male and female animals. The high dose should be sufficiently high to induce toxic responses in test animals; the low dose should not induce toxic responses in test animals, and the intermediate dose should be sufficiently high to elicit minimal toxic effects in test animals (such as alterations in enzyme levels or slight decreases in body weight gains). A contemporaneous control group is also required.

Ophthalmological examination, haematology profiles, clinical chemistry tests, and urinalyses should be performed.

All animals should be subject to complete gross necropsy, including determining gross organ weight, and microscopic examination of all major organs and lymphoid tissue.

Further reading

CHMP. Guidance on acute toxicity. Questions and answers on the withdrawal of the 'note for guidance on single dose toxicity'. 2010. Available at: ℘ http://www.ema.europa.eu/docs/en_GB/document_library/Scientific_guideline/2010/07/WC500094590.pdf

FDA. Guidance on subacute toxicity. Available at: ℘ http://www.fda.gov/Food/GuidanceComplianceRegulatoryInformation/GuidanceDocuments/FoodIngredientsandPackaging/Redbook/ucm078345.htm

Chapter 3.14

Studies: objectives, design, conduct, and analysis

Overview

Clinical trials should be designed, conducted, and analysed according to sound scientific principles to achieve their objectives; and should be reported appropriately.

ICH E6 GCP outlines some important principles should be followed in planning the objectives, design, conduct, analysis and reporting of a clinical trial. The ICH E8 document 'General Considerations for Clinical Trials' describes internationally accepted principles and practices in the conduct of both individual clinical trials and overall development strategy for new medicinal products.

Objectives

As per ICH E6, the objectives of the study should be clearly stated. They may include exploratory or confirmatory characterization of safety and/or efficacy and/or assessment of pharmacokinetic parameters, and pharmacological, physiological, and biochemical effects.

Design

The appropriate study design should be chosen to provide the desired information. The following must be taken into account:
- Appropriate comparators should be used.
- Sample size should be appropriate.
- Primary and secondary endpoints, and plans for their analyses, should be clearly stated (ICH E9).
- The methods of monitoring adverse events should be described (see ICH E3).
- The protocol should specify procedures for the follow-up of patients who stop treatment prematurely.
  Specific attention must be placed on:
- Selection of subjects.
- Selection of control group.
- Number of subjects.
- Response variables.
- Methods to minimize bias.

Selection of subjects
- As a general principle trial subjects should not participate concurrently in more than one clinical trial, but there can be justified exceptions.
- In general, women of childbearing potential should be using highly effective contraception to participate in clinical trials (ICH M3).
- For male subjects, potential hazards of drug exposure in the trial to their sexual partners or resulting progeny should be considered.

Selection of control group

Trials should have an adequate control group. The choice of the comparator depends on, among other things, the objective of the trial. Comparisons may be made with placebo, no treatment, active controls, or of different doses of the drug under investigation.

Number of subjects

Statistical assessments of sample size should be based on:
- The expected magnitude of the treatment effect.
- The variability of the data.
- The specified probability of error.
- The desire for information or subsets of the population or secondary endpoints.

Response variables

- A primary endpoint should reflect clinically relevant effects and is typically selected based on the principal objective of the study.
- Endpoints and the plan for their analysis should be prospectively specified in the protocol.
- Surrogate endpoints may be used as primary endpoints when appropriate.

Methods to minimize bias

The protocol should specify methods of allocation to treatment groups and blinding (ICH E9 and E10).

Randomization

In conducting a controlled trial, randomized allocation is the preferred means of assuring comparability of test groups and minimizing the possibility of selection bias.

Blinding

Blinding is an important means of reducing or minimizing the risk of biased study outcomes.

Compliance

Methods used to evaluate patient usage of the test drug should be specified in the protocol and the actual usage documented.

Conduct

The study should be conducted according to the GCP principles outlined in ICH E6.

Adherence to the study protocol is essential. A clear description of the rationale for any modification should be provided in a protocol amendment. Timely adverse event reporting during a study is essential.

Analysis

The study protocol should have a specified analysis plan that is appropriate for the objectives and design of the study.

A description of the statistical methods to be employed, including timing of any planned interim analysis, should be included in the protocol (ICH E3, ICH E6 and ICH E9).

The results of a clinical trial should be analysed in accordance with the plan prospectively stated in the protocol, and all deviations from the plan should be indicated in the study report. Safety data should be collected for all clinical trials, appropriately tabulated and with adverse events classified according to their seriousness and their likely causal relationship (ICH E2A).

Reporting

Clinical study reports should be adequately documented according to ICH E3.

Further reading

ICH Topic E8. General considerations for clinical trials. ℘ http://www.ich.org

Populations for exploratory studies and planning of exploratory studies

Populations for exploratory studies

Exploratory studies have non-therapeutic objectives and are conducted for the purpose of generating pharmacology data. As such they are traditionally conducted in healthy volunteers.

In certain indications, however, they may provide valuable data when these are conducted in patients. One example is in hypertension, where early studies conducted in subjects with mild hypertension may provide valuable early evidence on the PD effect of an investigational agent.

In HIV, oncology, and certain immunological indications, where agents may carry a significant level of toxicity, it is mandated that exploratory studies should be conducted in the patient population.

Phase I studies may not necessarily be blinded, or blinding may be difficult to achieve. For example, administration of a monoclonal antibody may result in significant symptoms related to cytokine release.

Planning of exploratory studies

Key to the planning of successful exploratory clinical studies is the clinical trial application (CTA) package.

This includes pre-clinical data on:
- Pharmacological basis of principal effects (mechanism of action).
- Dose–response or concentration–response relationships and duration of action.
- Systemic general pharmacology, including pharmacological effects on major organ systems and physiological responses.
- Studies of absorption, distribution, metabolism, and excretion.

Regulatory consultation

The FDA offers extensive guidance on IND submission. This includes the possibility of pre-IND consultation. The basis of the pre-IND consultation is to determine what aspects of the following package are required for the IND submission:
- *Animal pharmacology and toxicology studies:* preclinical data to permit an assessment as to whether the product is reasonably safe for initial testing in humans. Also included are any previous experience with the drug in humans (often foreign use).
- *Manufacturing information:* information pertaining to the composition, manufacturer, stability, and controls used for manufacturing the drug substance and the drug product. This information is assessed to ensure that the company can adequately produce and supply consistent batches of the drug.
- *Clinical protocols and investigator information:* detailed protocols for proposed clinical studies to assess whether the initial-phase trials will expose subjects to unnecessary risks. Also, information on the qualifications of clinical investigators—professionals (generally physicians) who oversee the administration of the experimental

compound—to assess whether they are qualified to fulfill their clinical trial duties. Finally, commitments to obtain informed consent from the research subjects, to obtain review of the study by an IRB, and to adhere to the investigational new drug regulations.

Similar pre-CTA consultation meetings exist with Health Canada, and scientific advice can be obtained from country agencies within Europe (see Chapter 4.2).

Further reading

EMEA. General considerations for clinical trials (1998). Available at: ℘ http://www.ema.europa.eu/docs/en_GB/document_library/Scientific_guideline/2009/09/WC500002877.pdf

FDA. Guidance on IND submission. Available at: ℘ http://www.fda.gov/Drugs/DevelopmentApprovalProcess/HowDrugsareDevelopedandApproved/ApprovalApplications/InvestigationalNewDrugINDApplication/default.htm

Pharmacodynamic endpoints

Pharmacodynamic endpoints

Pharmacodynamics describes the action of a medicinal product on the body, following administration—what the drug does to the body (as opposed to pharmacokinetics—what the body does to the drug). Pharmacodynamic endpoints are outcome measures that allow capture of the potential clinical benefit of a medicinal product. An endpoint may be a quantitative measurement representing a specific parameter, a binary clinical outcome indicating whether an event has occurred, or a time to occurrence of an event of interest. In the context of a confirmatory clinical trial, an endpoint can be defined as a measurement that allows us to decide whether the null hypothesis should be accepted or rejected.

Clinical trials

Clinical development

Clinical trials generally seek to determine the impact of a medicinal product on a defined population of patients. In order to assess this activity, pharmacodynamic endpoints are selected according to the objectives of the study. Endpoints should be:
- Capable of accurately and reliably answering the principle trial objectives.
- Clinically meaningful.
- Should relate to the disease process.
- Clearly defined and justified in the clinical trial protocol.
- Practical to collect.

Clinical and surrogate endpoints
- A clinical endpoint is defined as a characteristic or variable that reflects how a patient feels, functions, or survives.
- A surrogate endpoint is a biomarker intended to substitute for a clinical endpoint.
- A surrogate endpoint is expected to reliably predict clinical benefit (or harm, or lack of benefit or harm) based on epidemiological, therapeutic, pathophysiological, or other scientific evidence.
- A biomarker is a characteristic that is objectively measured and evaluated as an indicator of normal biological processes, pathogenic processes, or pharmacological responses to a therapeutic intervention.

Primary and secondary endpoints

Endpoints can be classified as primary and secondary endpoints. Primary endpoints measure outcomes that will answer the most important question being asked of the study. There is generally only one primary endpoint, and this endpoint should provide the most clinically relevant and convincing evidence of drug activity (e.g. overall survival). Secondary endpoints seek to establish other pertinent questions and are generally supportive measurements related to the primary objective (e.g. response rate, duration of response, health-related quality of life). The number of secondary variables should be limited and an explanation of their relative importance and role in interpretation of the study results should be included in the study protocol.

Composite endpoints

Often a clinical trial will have a single primary endpoint based on just one outcome measure. However, some clinical trials have primary endpoints consisting of multiple outcome measures, so-called composite endpoints. A composite endpoint consisting of a number of individual endpoints means that more outcome events will be captured and this may mean fewer patients are required in the clinical study. The components of the composite should be based on biological plausibility, and be clinically meaningful and of similar importance to the patient.

Further reading

ICH (1997). ICH harmonised tripartite guideline. General considerations for clinical trials. E8. Available at: ℘ http://www.ich.org/fileadmin/Public_Web_Site/ICH_Products/Guidelines/Efficacy/ E8/Step4/E8_Guideline.pdf

ICH (1998). ICH harmonised tripartite guideline. Statistical principles for clinical trials. E9. Available at: ℘ http://www.ich.org/fileadmin/Public_Web_Site/ICH_Products/Guidelines/Efficacy/E9/Step4/ E9_Guideline.pdf

Bioavailability and bioequivalence

Bioavailability (F)

Bioavailability is defined as the proportion of an administered dose of a drug that reaches the systemic circulation, normally expressed as a percentage. For IV administered drugs, the bioavailability is 100%. For oral drugs, only a proportion of the drug will reach the systemic circulation due to incomplete absorption and/or first pass metabolism. Absolute bioavailability compares the bioavailability of an IV administered drug to the bioavailability of a non-IV administered drug. Relative bioavailability compares the bioavailability of two non-IV administered drugs (e.g. tablet vs. oral solution).

Generic medicinal products

The activity of a drug is determined by its chemical concentration at the site of action. This may be the drug itself or an active metabolite. Rather than repeat the evidence for safety and efficacy of an innovator drug, generics abridge to these data with proof that the new formulation has the same bioavailability as the innovator product. The definition for a 'generic medicinal product' is found in Directive 2001/83/EC, Article 10(2)(b), and a generic medicinal product shall mean a medicinal product that has the same qualitative and quantitative composition in active substances and the same pharmaceutical form as the reference medicinal product, and whose bioequivalence with the reference medicinal product has been demonstrated by appropriate bioavailability studies.

Bioequivalence study

For most generics, potential formulation differences are tested in normal healthy volunteers in a randomized two-period, two-sequence cross-over designed study. Subjects are administered single doses of 'test' and 'reference' product and the test medicinal product should be representative of the product to be marketed. The two treatments are separated by a washout period, which must be sufficiently long to ensure drug concentrations in the next period are below the lower limit of bioanalytical detection (at least 5 elimination half-lives). Studies are normally carried out with a minimum of 12 healthy subjects. However, it may be necessary to perform the study with patients if there are safety concerns.

The test conditions should be standardized, e.g. with respect to food, and a sufficient number of samples are required to adequately describe the plasma concentration time profile. The evaluation of bioequivalence should usually be based on the measured concentrations of the parent compound, using a validated bioanalytical method. To determine bioequivalence, the parameters to be analysed are AUC (the area under the concentration time curve, reflecting the extent of exposure) and Cmax (the maximum plasma concentration or peak exposure, which is influenced by the absorption rate). Pharmacokinetic parameters should be analysed using ANOVA. The assessment of bioequivalence is based upon 90%

confidence intervals for the ratio of the population geometric means (test/reference) for AUC and Cmax. Two medicinal products containing the same active substance are considered bioequivalent if their bioavailabilities (rate and extent) lie within acceptable predefined limits. These limits are set to ensure comparable in vivo performance, i.e. similarity in terms of safety and efficacy and the proposed limits should be pre-specified in the study protocol. The predefined limits are specified in Table 3.17.1.

Table 3.17.1 Predefined limits for bioavailabilities

Characteristic	Acceptable limits 90% confidence interval	
	AUC	Cmax
Standard	80.00–125.00%	80.00–125.00%
Narrow therapeutic index drugs	90.00–111.11%	90.00–111.11%*
Highly variable drugs	80.00–125.00%	69.84–143.19% (maximum range**)

* When Cmax is of importance for safety, efficacy, or drug level monitoring.

** The extent of widening depends on the within-subject variability.

Special and complex bioequivalence problems include inhaled drugs, drugs with a narrow therapeutic margin, highly variable drugs, transdermal patches, suppositories, modified release, fixed dose combinations, or drugs whose active is a plasma constituent (e.g. slow release potassium).

Biosimilars

A biosimilar medicine is a drug that is similar to a biological medicine that has already been authorized (the biological reference). Large biological molecules are difficult to copy. Even if the primary, secondary, and tertiary structure of a biological molecule is correct, modifications such as phosphorylation and glycosylation may alter function. Comparability studies are generally needed to generate evidence substantiating the similar nature, in terms of quality, safety, and efficacy, of the new similar biological medicinal product and the chosen reference medicinal product authorized in the Community. The first biosimilar medicinal product was authorized in Europe in 2006 (Somatrophin).

Further reading

EMA. Guideline on the investigation of bioequivalence (2010). Available at: ℘ http://www.emea.europa.eu/docs/en_GB/document_library/Scientific_guideline/2010/01/WC500070039.pdf

EMA. Guideline on similar biological medicinal products containing biotechnology-derived proteins as active substance: non-clinical and clinical issues (2006). Available at: ℘ http://www.ema.europa.eu/docs/en_GB/document_library/Scientific_guideline/2009/09/WC500003920.pdf

EMA. Guideline on similar biological medicinal products (2005). Available at: ℘ http://www.emea.europa.eu/docs/en_GB/document_library/Scientific_guideline/2009/09/WC500003517.pdf

Evaluation of safety and tolerability

Overview

In all clinical trials evaluation of safety and tolerability constitutes an important element. ICH Topic E9: Statistical principles for clinical trials provides guidance on capturing safety and tolerability data in clinical trials and is summarized below.

Early exploratory phases are only sensitive to frank expressions of toxicity. Later phases can help characterize the safety and tolerability profile of a drug more fully.

The methods chosen to evaluate the safety and tolerability of a drug will depend on a number of factors, including:

- Knowledge of the adverse effects of closely related drugs.
- Information from non-clinical and earlier clinical trials.
- Pharmacodynamic/pharmacokinetic properties of the particular drug.
- Mode of administration.
- Type of subjects to be studied.
- Duration of the trial.

Laboratory tests, vital signs, and clinical adverse events form the main body of the safety and tolerability data. The occurrence of serious adverse events and treatment discontinuations due to adverse events are particularly important to register (ICH E2A and ICH E3). The use of a common adverse event dictionary is particularly important.

Set of subjects to be evaluated and presentation of data

- For the overall safety and tolerability assessment, the set of subjects to be summarized is usually defined as those subjects who received at least one dose of the investigational drug.
- All adverse events should be reported, whether or not they are considered to be related to treatment. All available data in the study population should be accounted for in the evaluation.
- In situations when there is a substantial background noise of signs and symptoms, one should consider ways of accounting for this in the estimation of risk for different adverse events. One such method is to make use of the 'treatment emergent' concept in which adverse events are recorded only if they emerge or worsen relative to pretreatment baseline.

Statistical evaluation

Although some specific adverse effects can usually be anticipated, the range of possible, and new and unforeseeable adverse effects is very large.

This underlies the statistical difficulties associated with the evaluation of safety and tolerability of drugs. Therefore, conclusive information from confirmatory clinical trials is unusual.

In most trials, the safety and tolerability implications are best addressed by applying descriptive statistical methods to the data, supplemented by calculation of confidence intervals wherever this aids interpretation. It is also valuable to make use of graphical presentations in which patterns of adverse events are displayed both within treatment groups and within subjects.

The calculation of p-values is sometimes useful either as an aid to evaluating a specific difference of interest, or as a 'flagging' device applied to a large number of safety and tolerability variables to highlight differences worth further attention.

Laboratory data should be subjected to both a quantitative analysis, e.g. evaluation of treatment means, and a qualitative analysis where counting of numbers above or below certain thresholds are calculated.

If hypothesis tests are used, the type II error is of most concern.

In the majority of trials, investigators are seeking to establish that there are no clinically unacceptable differences in safety and tolerability compared with either a comparator drug or a placebo. The use of confidence intervals is preferred in this situation.

Integrated summary

The safety and tolerability properties of a drug are commonly summarized across trials continuously during an investigational product's development and, in particular, at the time of a marketing application. The usefulness of this summary, however, is dependent on adequate and well-controlled individual trials with high data quality.

The overall usefulness of a drug is always a question of balance between risk and benefit, and in a single trial, such a perspective could also be considered, even if the assessment of risk/benefit usually is performed in the summary of the entire clinical trial programme.

Further reading

ICH Topic E9 (1998). Statistical principles for clinical trials. CPMP/ICH/363/96. Available at: ☞ http://www.emea.europa.eu/docs/en_GB/document_library/Scientific_guideline/2009/09/WC500002928.pdf

Chapter 3.19

Hypersensitivity reactions

Overview

Both immune- and non-immune-mediated drug reactions occur. Amongst immune-mediated drug reactions, the type I–IV classification is followed.

Type I reactions

These are IgE dependent reactions that lead to urticaria, angioedema, and anaphylaxis. Typical drugs that result in Type I reactions include therapeutic peptides.

Type II reactions

These are cytotoxic hypersensitivity reactions resulting in haemolysis and purpura. Typical drugs resulting in Type II reactions include penicillins, sulphonamides, cephalosporins, and rifampicin.

Type III reactions

These are immune complex mediated reactions leading to vasculitis, serum sickness and an urticarial rash. Drugs which are known to be associated with immune complex reactions include quinine, salicylates, and sulphonamides.

Type IV reactions

These reactions are not dose-dependent and usually begin 7–20 days after initiation of therapy, they are the commonest type of hypersensitivity drug reaction. Only a minority of cutaneous drug reactions, however, have a demonstrable link to IgE, with <5% having anti-drug antibodies.

Drug-induced angioedema

Acquired angioedema is commonly reported in response to angiotensin-converting-enzyme (ACE) inhibition, less often with angiotensin II receptor blockers (ARBS). With respect to ACE inhibitors this may be related to changes in the metabolism of bradykinin, although this does not explain why ARBS lead to angioedema. Urticarial angioedema is seen with aspirin and non-steroidal anti-inflammatory drug (NSAID) use.

Investigation of hypersensitivity

- Skin biopsy may demonstrate eosinophilic or neutrophilic infiltration.
- Full blood count may reveal raised peripheral blood eosinophil count, leukopaenia or thrombocytopaenia.
- Special attention should be drawn to associated abnormalities in liver function tests.
- Antibody/immunoserology testing may be useful.
- Patch testing is of very limited value, and may actually be dangerous in the case of previous severe cutaneous skin reaction.
- Urinalysis may be useful where there is suspected underlying vasculitis.

Hypersensitivity reactions in the context of a clinical trial

Whilst minor injection site rashes may be seen in as many as 5–10% of subjects given therapeutic proteins subcutaneously, serious hypersensitivity reactions are much rarer,

For this reason, in studies up to phase IIb, when only perhaps a few hundred patients or more have been exposed to a new agent, serious hypersensitivity may not become apparent.

Idiopathic hypersensitivity reactions may indeed not become apparent until after phase III, once exposure to a drug expands because it has been launched on the market.

Monitoring comes largely from healthcare professional reports of adverse drug reactions, such as the Yellow Card system used in the UK, although these are imperfect, only perhaps recording around 5% of adverse drug reactions.

Further reading

Pitcher WJ (2007). *Drug hypersensitivity*. Basel: Karger.

Drug–drug interactions

Overview

Drug–drug interactions may be pharmacokinetic or pharmacodynamic, which may or may not lead to differences in the clinical responses seen compared with when the individual drugs are administered alone.

Characterization of drug–drug interactions

Altered absorption

Due to chelation or complex formation (cholestyramine and warfarin), prokinetic effects (metaclopramide reducing paracetamol absorption), pH changes (H2 blockade reducing absorption of ketoconazole).

Altered distribution

Competition between two drugs for the same protein-binding site may lead to increased free concentration of the lower affinity drug. This is particularly important with respect to protein-bound drugs with relatively low affinity such as warfarin.

Altered transport

Drugs may compete for the same active transporters. One example being quinidine and digoxin, where both compete for the *MDR-1* gene encoded P-glycoprotein, such that quinidine increases plasma concentration of digoxin.

Induction/inhibition

CYP450 induction/inhibition is crucially important in assessing potential drug–drug interactions. A number of databases exist listing known P450 inhibitors and inducers; the link for one such site is provided.

Altered excretion

Changes in urinary pH and competition for renal anion and cation transporters may impact on drug excretion. One prime example is probenecid, which reduces renal excretion of penicillins.

Interactions are likely to be particularly important when:
• Elimination of a drug occurs primarily through a single metabolic pathway.
• A drug is a potent inhibitor or inducer of a drug-metabolizing enzyme.
• One or both of the interacting drugs has a steep dose–response curve.
• One or both of the interacting drugs has a narrow therapeutic range.
• Inhibition of the primary metabolic enzyme or induction of a secondary metabolic enzyme results in diversion of the drug into an alternative metabolic pathway that generates a metabolite having toxic or modified pharmacodynamic activity.
• A drug has non-linear pharmacokinetics or when the interaction results in conversion from linear to non-linear pharmacokinetics.

In vitro testing for interactions

- *Liver microsomal screening:* allows for testing for P450, flavin containing mono-oxygenases, glucuronyl transferase, and hydrolase interactions.
- *Whole cell models:* whole cell models exist for liver metabolism, using liver slices, which preserve architecture and for intestinal absorption, and methods now also exist for culturing human hepatocytes. These can be combined with pharmacological probes with known interaction profiles.

In vivo clinical testing

- Cross-over or parallel group designs can be considered for drug–drug interaction studies depending on predicted half-life/washout period for the agent under investigation, and whether single or multiple dosing is required (is the agent under study predicted to require single or chronic dosing?).
- The population for a drug interaction study depends on the objectives, initially, a healthy cohort with restrictive eligibility criteria may be considered. Later the eligibility will be expanded, then patients who meet the criteria of the label will be recruited, and finally those with polymorphisms likely to predispose to possible drug–drug interactions may be studied.
- Route of administration should be that which is intended for the clinic, the dose used should be the maximal intended, and the dosing interval the shortest intended.
- Endpoints should include PK endpoints such as AUC, the peak concentration (Cmax), the time to peak concentration (t-max), the trough concentration (Cmin), the clearance (Cl), the volume of distribution (Vd), and the elimination half-life ($t_{1/2}$).
- Relevant PD endpoints should be included, for instance when mechanisms may be complementary and any interaction not necessarily completely accounted for by PK alone.

Drug–disease interaction

- Drug–disease interactions may be pharmacokinetic or pharmacodynamic.
- Diseases associated with low plasma proteins, such as liver disease, malabsorption, or nephrotic syndrome may lead to increased free levels of drugs, which are highly protein bound, such as warfarin or phenytoin.
- Low renal clearance may be associated with accumulation of drugs, which are predominantly renally excreted; these include sulphonylureas such as glibenclamide, antibiotics such as gentamicin, and agents from other drug classes such as allopurinol.
- Other drugs may impact negatively on co-morbidities. One obvious example is the use of beta blockade, which may worsen symptoms of wheeze and shortness of breath in patients with underlying asthma, or exacerbate erectile dysfunction in those with pre-existing difficulties.

Accounting for drug–disease interaction in the clinical trial programme

In vitro data and data from healthy volunteer PK/PD studies will provide important clues as to whether significant hepatic, renal, or cardiac dysfunction will impact significantly on effects of the investigational agent in the target population.

If significant potential risk is identified, then a targeted drug–disease interaction study can be considered. Examples may include a PK/PD study in patients with renal impairment, or one in patients with low plasma proteins if a potential agent undergoes significant protein binding.

Further reading

P450 interaction table. Available at: ℘ http://medicine.iupui.edu/clinpharm/ddis/

Health Canada Guidelines on drug–drug interaction studies. Available at: ℘ http://www.hc-sc. gc.ca/dhp-mps/prodpharma/applic-demande/guide-ld/interactions/drug_medl_int-eng.php

Ethics in research: basic principles, Declaration of Helsinki, and Council for International Organizations of Medical Sciences

Overview

All research involving human subjects should be conducted in accordance with three basic ethical principles:
• Respect for persons.
• Beneficence.
• Justice.

It is generally agreed that these principles guide the conscientious preparation of proposals for scientific studies.
• Respect for persons incorporates at least two fundamental ethical considerations, namely:
  • Respect for autonomy.
  • Protection of persons with impaired or diminished autonomy.
• Beneficence refers to the ethical obligation to maximize benefits and to minimize harm. This principle gives rise to norms requiring that the risks of research be reasonable in the light of the expected benefits, that the research design is sound, and that the investigators be competent both to conduct the research and to safeguard the welfare of the research subjects.
• Justice refers to the ethical obligation to treat each person in accordance with what is morally right and proper, to give each person what is due to him or her. In the ethics of research involving human subjects the principle refers primarily to *distributive justice*, which requires the equitable distribution of both the burdens and the benefits of participation in research.

The first international instrument on the ethics of medical research, the Nuremberg Code, set out basic principles to be observed when conducting research involving human subjects and subsequently formed the basis for comprehensive international guidelines on medical research, such as the Declaration of Helsinki.

The Declaration of Helsinki

The Declaration of Helsinki was adopted by the World Medical Association in 1964 as 'a statement of ethical principles to provide guidance to physicians and other participants in medical research involving human subjects.'[1] It is the fundamental document in the field of ethics in biomedical research and has influenced the formulation of international, regional, and national legislation and codes of conduct. It has been amended six times, the most recent version being in 2008. It is a comprehensive international statement of the ethics of research involving human subjects. It sets out ethical guidelines for physicians engaged in both clinical and non-clinical biomedical research.

1 Reproduced from the Declaration of Helsinki, 'Ethical Principles for Medical Research Involving Human Subjects', last amended 2008, with permission from the World Medical Association.

Council for International Organizations of Medical Sciences

Most recently, the Council for International Organizations and Medical Sciences (CIOMS) produced detailed guidelines on the implementation of the principles outlined in the Declaration of Helsinki. The CIOMS guidelines address the areas given in Box 3.21.1.

Box 3.21.1 Summary of CIOMS guidelines

1. Ethical justification and scientific validity of biomedical research involving human beings.
2. Ethical review committees.
3. Ethical review of externally sponsored research.
4. Individual informed consent.
5. Obtaining informed consent: essential information for prospective research subjects.
6. Obtaining informed consent: obligations of sponsors and investigators.
7. Inducement to participate.
8. Benefits and risks of study participation.
9. Special limitations on risk when research involves individuals who are not capable of giving informed consent.
10. Research in populations and communities with limited resources.
11. Choice of control in clinical trials.
12. Equitable distribution of burdens and benefits in the selection of groups of subjects in research.
13. Research involving vulnerable persons.
14. Research involving children.
15. Research involving individuals who by reason of mental or behavioural disorders are not capable of giving adequately informed consent.
16. Women as research subjects.
17. Pregnant women as research participants.
18. Safeguarding confidentiality.
19. Right of injured subjects to treatment and compensation.
20. Strengthening capacity for ethical and scientific review, and biomedical research.
21. Ethical obligation of external sponsors to provide healthcare services.

Further reading

International Ethical Guidelines for Biomedical Research Involving Human Subjects. Prepared by the Council for International Organizations of Medical Sciences (CIOMS) in collaboration with the World Health Organization (WHO). Geneva: CIOMS, 2002.

World Medical Association. Declaration of Helsinki: ethical principles for medical research involving human subjects. Available at: ✆ www.wma.net/e/policy/b3.htm

The Council for International Organizations and Medical Sciences (CIOMS). Guidelines on Ethics of Clinical Trials. *Proc Am Thorac Soc* 2007; **4**, 176–9.

Disease models

Overview

Animal disease models exist for a number of chronic conditions, particularly metabolic and cardiovascular diseases. They provide valuable pre-clinical information to support progression of agents into human clinical studies.

Examples of disease models by indication are described in Table 3.22.1.

Table 3.22.1 Examples of disease models by indication

Indication	Relevant models
Cardiovascular disease	Spontaneously hypertensive heart failure (SHHF)
Fasting hyperglycaemia	GK, Obese Prone Rat (OP-CD), Obese Resistant Rat (OR-CD), ZDF, ZSF1
Hypercholesterolaemia	Dahl/SS, SHHF, SHR, SHROB, Stroke Prone SHR, ZDF, ZSF1, Zucker
Hyperinsulinaemia	Dahl/SS, GK, Obese Prone Rat (OP-CD), Obese Resistant Rat (OR-CD), SHHF, SHR, SHROB, Stroke Prone SHR, ZDF, ZSF1, Zucker
Hypertension	Dahl/SS, FHH, Obese Prone Rat (OP-CD), Obese Resistant Rat (OR-CD), SHR, SHHF, SHROB, Stroke Prone SHR, ZSF1
Hypertriglyceridaemia	Dahl/SS, SHHF, Obese Prone Rat (OP-CD), Obese Resistant Rat (OR-CD), SHR, SHROB, Stroke Prone SHR, ZDF, ZSF1, Zucker
Insulin resistance	Dahl/SS, GK, Obese Prone Rat (OP-CD), Obese Resistant Rat (OR-CD), SHHF, SHR, SHROB, Stroke Prone SHR, ZDF, ZSF1, Zucker
Nephropathy	Dahl/SS, GK, SHHF, SHROB, Stroke Prone SHR, ZDF, ZSF1, Zucker
Type 2 diabetes	GK, SHHF, ZDF, ZSF1
Obesity	Obese Prone Rat (OP-CD), SHHF, SHROB, ZDF, ZSF1, Zucker
Polycystic kidney disease	PCK

From: Charles River Laboratories. Disease models. Available at: ⌖ http://www.criver.com/en-US/ProdServ/ByType/ResModOver/diseasemodels/Pages/diseasemodelsbyindication.aspx

Models also exist for pre-clinical studies of agents with potential oncology indications. The National Cancer Institute supports a website acting as a repository for animal cancer models. The site eMICE offers a range of information about generation of models by organ and tumour type.

Further reading

Cardiovascular/metabolic medicine disease models:

Charles River Laboratories, Disease models. Available at: ℘ http://www.criver.com/en-US/ ProdServ/ByType/ResModOver/diseasemodels/Pages/diseasemodelsbyindication.aspx

eMICE:

eMICE: Electronic Models Information, Communication, and Education, National Cancer Institue, US National Institutes of Health. Available at: ℘ http://emice.nci.nih.gov/

Chapter 3.23

Biomarkers

Biomarkers

Biomarkers are playing an increasingly important role in drug discovery by helping to streamline clinical development. 'Biomarker' is a broad term and is defined as a characteristic that is objectively measured and evaluated as an indicator of normal biological processes, pathogenic processes, or pharmacological responses to a therapeutic intervention. A prognostic biomarker provides information about a patients overall clinical outcome, regardless of the therapy. A predictive biomarker identifies subpopulations of patients who are most likely to respond to a specific therapy or medicinal product. A predictive biomarker can be a target for therapy. Biomarkers have a variety of uses in drug development:

• Indicator of disease prognosis.
• Diagnostic tool.
• Proof of concept studies.
• Phase 0 studies (administration of subtherapeutic microdoses).
• Provision of data for PK/PD modelling.
• Dose selection/dose ranging.
• Staging/classification of disease.
• Patient stratification and candidate selection for clinical studies.
• Predict or measure clinical response to an intervention (surrogate endpoint).

Surrogate endpoints

A biomarker that is intended to replace a clinical endpoint is called a surrogate endpoint (a clinical endpoint is defined as a characteristic or variable that reflects how a patient feels, functions, or survives). The surrogate endpoint must effectively and consistently predict clinical benefit or the lack of clinical benefit. The process of linking a surrogate endpoint to a clinical endpoint is referred to as qualification. Qualification of biomarkers for regulatory acceptance is both time-consuming and resource intensive. Consortiums/partnerships have been launched to promote the discovery, development, validation, and regulatory acceptance of biomarkers. Biomarkers, which are potentially good candidates as surrogate endpoints are shown in Table 3.23.1 (the Bradford Hill Criteria).

Table 3.23.1 Bradford Hill Criteria

Biomarker characteristic	Description
Strength	Strong association between outcome of interest and the marker
Consistency/coherence	The relationship is consistent between different situations and individuals and the natural history of the disease
Specificity	Disease specific indicator
Temporality	Observed changes occur in parallel
Dose responsiveness	A biological gradient is observed—increasing exposure to a therapy results in increasing effects on the disease and the marker
Plausibility	Strong scientific rationale links the marker to the disease process and therapeutic intervention
Experimental evidence	The results seen with a therapeutic intervention supports the rationale for the association

Further reading

Biomarkers Definitions Working Group. Biomarkers and surrogate endpoints: preferred definitions and conceptual framework. *Clin Pharmacol Therapeut* 2001; **69**(3): 89–95.

EMA. Qualification of novel methodologies for drug development: guidance to applicants. Doc. Ref. EMEA/CHMP/SAWP/72894/2008 Corr1. Available at: ℜ http://www.rsihata.com/updateguidance/emea/2009/7289408en.pdf

Pharmacogenetics

Overview

There has been a rapid development regarding our understanding of the genetics behind inter-individual differences in drug response.

- In practice, genetic variations are demonstrated by the identification of single nucleotide polymorphisms (SNPs), insertions/deletions, and gene copy number variation (CNV).
- With respect to PK aspects, the highest abundance of genetic polymorphism is registered at the level of drug metabolism where ~40% of phase I metabolism of clinically used drugs is catalyzed by enzymes with polymorphisms known to have marked impact on in vivo function.
- Well-known variable enzymes in this respect are the cytochrome P450 enzymes CYP2D6, CYP2C9, and CYP2C19.
- When considering phase II enzymes, the genetic variability of UDP-glucuronosyltransferases, N-acetyltransferase-2, and some methyltransferases have been shown to play a role in the inter-individual variability in PK.
- Where significant polymorphisms have been identified in authorized products, metabolizing enzymes account for 80% of pharmacogenetic labelling.
- At present, an increasing fraction of drugs selected for development are metabolized by enzymes, for which there is very little knowledge on the impact of pharmacogenetics.
- New technologies, like the whole genome-wide association studies (GWAS) methodology, have already been shown to be informative regarding the genetic basis for inter-individual differences in drug distribution and adverse reactions, and are already to some extent incorporated in clinical development programmes.
- With respect to inclusion in studies, in vitro P450 panels have an important role in pre-clinical work up of compounds. Any suggestion of a 2D6/C9/C1 interaction then drives specific in vivo drug–drug interaction studies, and genetic sampling is encouraged in phase IIb and phase III for all new programmes now.
- Prospective collection of data allows for outliers in the case of either drug metabolism, therapeutic response, or adverse event profile to be analysed for specific genetic polymorphisms.
- Examples of interactions where prospective collection of pharmacogenetic data has proved useful include CYP2C19 polymorphisms and response to clopidogrel, and HLA B5701 and abacavir hypersensitivity. In the case of abacavir this has led to the development of a specific bench test prior to starting therapy.

Further reading

EMA. Concept paper on the development of a guideline on the use of pharmacogenomic methodologies in the pharmacokinetic evaluation of medicinal products. Available at: ℘ http://www.ema.europa.eu/docs/en_GB/document_library/Scientific_guideline/2009/09/WC500003862.pdf

Mallal S, Phillips E, Carosi G, et al. (2008). HLA-B*5701 screening for hypersensitivity to abacavir. N Engl J Med; **358**(6): 568–79. Available at: ℘ http://www.nejm.org/doi/full/10.1056/NEJMoa0706135

Population pharmacokinetics

Overview

Traditional PK studies examine the effects of a small number of variables such as age, sex, disease, concomitant medication, etc., in a controlled study on the PK of a drug. The problem is that the small sample may not be representative of the population for which the drug is intended, or indeed the population for recruitment into phase III. Also small samples may miss factors such as genetic polymorphisms impacting on drug metabolism.

Population PK varies in that a much smaller number of PK samples are collected from each patient, but each patient, for instance in a phase III programme, contributes some PK data. This allows construction of a time concentration graph from thousands of pieces of data. A major advantage is that it therefore allows outliers to be detected, and their data can be examined for previously undiscovered factors, which impact on the time concentration curve.

A disadvantage, of course, is that population PK potentially requires the collection of thousands of extra samples, which may come from quite disparate phase IIb/III sites. This can incur significant extra cost.

Paediatric studies lend themselves particularly well to population PK, as sparse sampling is significantly less onerous for the subjects concerned. The technique is therefore recommended by regulatory authorities when considering the development of dosing regimens in children.

Further reading

EMA. Guideline on the role of pharmacokinetics in the development of medicinal products in the paediatric population. Available at: ℘ http://www.ema.europa.eu/docs/en_GB/document_library/Scientific_guideline/2009/09/WC500003066.pdf

Small molecules and biologicals: safety and pharmacology requirements

Overview

A number of guidelines govern safety pharmacology requirements for both small molecules and biologicals:

- S6: Preclinical Safety Evaluation of Biotechnology-Derived Pharmaceuticals.
- S7A: Safety Pharmacology Studies for Human Pharmaceuticals.
- S7B: The Non-Clinical Evaluation of the Potential for Delayed Ventricular Repolarization (QT Interval Prolongation) by Human Pharmaceuticals.
- E14: The Clinical Evaluation of QT/QTc Interval Prolongation and Proarrhythmic Potential for Non-Antiarrhythmic Drugs.

Special considerations for biologics

- The nature and size of the molecule may drive specific studies, e.g. very different studies may be required for monoclonals, vs. proteins, vs. enzymes/small peptides.
- The molecular target and degree of tissue expression may also drive specific studies—different studies are likely to be needed, e.g. for a peptide directed against a tumour antigen vs. a white cell surface receptor vs. a growth factor.
- A biological may also be species specific. Classical examples include peptides directed against white cell surface receptors; certain species may be precluded from safety testing altogether due to toxicity, or may deliver results that are irrelevant in the context of human studies.
- Disposition and biological activity of the molecule is also important, limited vs. extensive distribution, presence or absence of CNS penetration, half-life vs. duration of effect, etc.
- Physicochemical characteristics of molecule, such as charge, lability/ stability and tendency to aggregate play a role in the type of studies chosen.
- Formulation, specifically scalability/differences with commercial process may be important when interpreting safety results.
- Development of specific assays, particularly for large molecules, is also crucial for the interpretation of PK data from safety studies.

Organ systems

Safety testing is designed to evaluate effects of an agent on first tier organ systems essential for sustaining life, the cardiovascular, nervous and respiratory systems, and second tier organ systems, such as the GI tract, renal, and immune systems.

Summary

Whilst a standard basket of safety pharmacology testing exists for small molecules, a pragmatic approach is crucial with respect to evaluating biologicals. Studies should be dictated by:
- Nature, biology, and species specificity of the molecule.
- Biology and expression of target.
- Availability of relevant model.
- Assay conditions and formulation components.
- Scientific rationale.
- Feasibility to conduct specific studies.

Section 4

Clinical development

Chapter 4.1

Requirements for licensing a new medicinal product

Medicinal product

The EC Directive 2001/83/EC defines a medicinal product as:
- Any substance or combination of substances presented as having properties for treating or preventing disease in human beings.
- Any substance or combination of substances that may be used in or administered to human beings, either with a view to restoring, correcting, or modifying physiological functions by exerting a pharmacological, immunological, or metabolic action, or to making a medical diagnosis.

EU legislation states that medicinal products for human use may only be placed on the market in the EU if a marketing authorization has been issued by the Community or by a competent authority of a member state. Therefore, for a medicine to be licensed, a marketing authorization application must be submitted to a national competent authority or the European Medicines Agency (EMA).

There are a number of different types of application procedure available and the procedure type depends on the nature of the active ingredient of the product and the proposed market area. The types of procedures are the centralized procedure, national procedure, decentralized procedure and the mutual recognition procedure. An MAA is usually submitted by a pharmaceutical company but anyone with the necessarily supporting data may apply. An MAA requires a fee, the level of which depends on the classification and complexity of the application.

Guidance

In the EU, there are a number of regulatory guidance documents which explain the requirements for licensing a new medicinal product. The European Union legislation in the pharmaceutical sector is compiled in Volume 1 of the publication *The Rules Governing Medicinal Products in the European Union*, Eudralex (Volume 1, *EU Pharmaceutical Legislation for Medicinal Products for Human Use*). Volume 2, *Pharmaceutical Legislation Notice to Applicants and Regulatory Guidelines Medicinal Products for Human Use*, provides very detailed information on the requirements for the submission of a marketing authorization application:
- Volume 2A: Procedures for marketing authorization.
- Volume 2B: Presentation and content of the dossier.
- Volume 2C: Regulatory guidelines.

The data package to support the application (administrative, quality, non-clinical and clinical) must comply with the common technical document (CTD [ICH M4]) format (the dossier).
- Following the submission of the dossier to a competent authority and before assessment, a validation step takes place where the dossier is checked against the requirements of the 'Notice to Applicants'.
- Omissions may be highlighted to the applicant or the application may be deemed invalid.

- Once validated, the application is then assessed by a multi-disciplinary team of professional assessors who may include clinicians, toxicologists, pharmacists, statisticians, and other scientific personnel.
- The assessment of an application normally follows a timetable with certain milestone dates at specific calendar days.
- Following the assessment of the quality, safety, and efficacy of the product, the assessment team reaches an initial conclusion regarding the application and a list of questions or request for further (supplementary) information is normally requested.
- The applicant has a set period time to respond in writing to the request and following receipt of the information the assessors review the data and draw final/further conclusions.
- In some circumstances and procedures, an applicant may withdraw their application from some or all member states involved.

Risk–benefit assessment

The assessment of the benefits and risks of a new drug is a complex process that requires the evaluation of a large amount of data. Expert judgement remains the cornerstone of the assessment task, and the evaluation must objectively achieve a satisfactory level of confidence that the quality, safety, and efficacy of the new medicinal product has been established. In arriving at a decision whether or not to grant a licence, independent expert advice may be sought on matters relating to quality, safety, and efficacy from medicines advisory bodies. In the UK, applications may be referred to advisory bodies such as Expert Advisory Groups (EAG) and the Commission on Human Medicines (CHM). In the centralized procedure, CHMP may request input from Scientific Advisory Groups (SAG).

At the end of the procedure the application is deemed by the competent authority to be either approvable or non-approvable. Some applications may only be approvable on the condition that certain follow-up measures are carried out by the applicant. For non-approvable decisions, an appeals process exists and applicants may appeal against a refusal by informing the authority in writing, within a defined time period.

Further reading

EudraLex. Volume 1, *Pharmaceutical Legislation Medicinal Products for Human Use*. Available at: ℗ http://ec.europa.eu/health/documents/eudralex/vol-1/index_en.htm

EudraLex. Volume 2, *Pharmaceutical Legislation Notice to Applicants and Regulatory Guidelines Medicinal Products for Human Use*. Available at: ℗ http://ec.europa.eu/health/documents/eudralex/vol-2/index_en.htm

Regulatory guidance

Scientific advice

The aim of scientific advice is to facilitate the development and availability of high-quality, effective and safe medicines. Scientific advice and protocol assistance can be sought from Regulatory Authorities regarding key areas of development of a medicinal product. Companies may request scientific advice either during the initial development of a medicinal product, before the submission of an MAA, or in the post-authorization setting. Seeking scientific advice is particularly important if a development plan deviates from the recommendations found in published regulatory scientific guidelines/pharmacopeia monographs, or if these documents are considered by the sponsor not to have sufficient detail. Specific scientific issues that may be addressed include quality, non-clinical, and clinical aspects of a development programme, pharmacovigilance plans and regulatory guidance.

Sponsors may seek scientific advice from the competent authorities of individual member states or from the EMA if pan-European advice is sought. Advice from the EMA is given by the CHMP on the recommendation of the Scientific Advice Working Party (SAWP). A fee, depending on the scope of the advice is usually payable. Fee reductions are available for designated orphan medicinal products, for the development of medicinal products for paediatric use and advanced therapy medicinal products, and for registered small and medium-sized enterprises.

The EMA also provides scientific advice in parallel with the United States FDA. It should be noted that scientific advice received from the EMA is not legally binding for either party with regards to any future application for a marketing authorization, and the advice may be adopted or rejected at the sponsor's discretion. However, seeking and adhering to scientific advice may reduce the likelihood of major objections being raised during an MAA, increasing the probability of a successful outcome.

In the USA, the FDA offers special protocol assessment (SPA) and agreement where protocols are assessed to determine whether they are adequate to meet scientific and regulatory requirements. SPA will not be provided after a study has commenced. Such assessment may include animal carcinogenicity, final product stability, and phase III trial clinical protocols and any agreement is considered binding. An SPA can be modified if the FDA and sponsor agree in writing to modify the protocol and such a change is intended to improve the study.

Regulatory guidelines

In Europe, the CHMP, in consultation with working parties and the competent authorities of EU member states, prepares scientific guidelines. The goal of these guidelines is to assist in the preparation of MAA for medicinal products for human use and to provide a basis for harmonization in the interpretation and application of Community Directives. The guidelines cover the detailed requirements for the demonstration of the quality, safety, and efficacy of medicinal products and are considered as complementary to other official documents, such as the European Pharmacopeia monographs.

CHMP clinical efficacy and safety guidelines cover the following topics (some covered by ICH topics):
- Clinical pharmacology and pharmacokinetics.
- Alimentary tract and metabolism.
- Blood and blood forming organs.
- Blood products (including biotech alternatives).
- Cardiovascular system.
- Dermatologicals.
- Genito-urinary system and sex hormones.
- Anti-infectives for systemic use.
- Antineoplastic and immunomodulating agents.
- Musculo-skeletal system.
- Nervous system.
- Respiratory system.
- General.
- Herbal medicinal products.
- Information on medicinal products.
- Radiopharmaceuticals and diagnostic agents.

In the USA, guidance documents are prepared by the FDA, representing the Agency's current thinking on a particular issue. Guidance documents do not bind the FDA or the sponsor to a specific course of action, and alternative approaches may be considered.

Further reading
EMA. Scientific guidelines. Available at: http://www.ema.europa.eu/ema/index.jsp?curl=pages/regulation/general/general_content_000043.jsp&mid=WC0b01ac05800240cb
FDA. Drugs: guidance, compliance and regulatory information. Available at: http://www.fda.gov/Drugs/GuidanceComplianceRegulatoryInformation/default.htm
ICH official website. http://www.ich.org/

Chapter 4.3

General principles of clinical trial protocols

Overview

Clinical trial protocols are designed according to principles established by the major regulatory agencies; because of harmonization of design principles, endpoint data, including adverse events can then be utilized in a range of submissions to regulators.

Major components

- *Summary page:* includes information on protocol number, version and date, phase of clinical investigation, name of investigational drug, IND or EUdract number, and authorized signatories.
- *Clinical study objectives:* incorporates the primary objectives of the study and key secondary endpoints.
- *Study design:* components of study design including blinding, treatment allocation, duration of intervention, etc.
- *Subject selection:* key inclusion and exclusion criteria.
- *Description of study drug:* includes formulation, administration, storage, manufacture, list of excipients, concomitant medications which should be avoided, and any rescue procedures in case of overdose/misdosing.
- *Study procedures:* includes list of any screening procedures required, on-drug investigations, any procedures to carry out around the time of drug administration. These are normally summarized as part of a time and events table.
- *Safety and effectiveness assessments:* what variables will be measured to determine both efficacy and acceptable safety and tolerability profile of the agent under investigation.
- *Adverse event reporting:* definition of serious and non-serious adverse events. Any specific criteria which may lead to a cessation in dosing or stopping the study completely.
- *Reporting requirements:* obligations of the investigator and the sponsor with respect to reporting suspected adverse events to regulatory authorities.
- *Statistical methods/data analysis:* this section contains a listing for the primary and other endpoints. It includes a section on how the study is powered, including statistical assumptions about what difference is expected for intervention vs. control in the primary endpoint.
- *Data and safety monitoring committee:* a phase III study may well incorporate a data and safety monitoring committee, and in the case of a phase III study, the make-up and operating rules of the DSMC are usually described here.
- *Data handling/records and retention:* description of how data will be stored, and rules about access to data.
- *Ethics approval:* a description of the need for ethical approval.
- *Informed consent:* a re-iteration of the rules around informed consent of subjects, and either in this section or as an appendix, a description/copy of the subject informed consent form.
- *References:* any references, e.g. the investigator's brochure/previous publications, which have been used to draw up the document.

Investigator's brochure

A protocol cannot contain all of the necessary information about an agent under clinical trial investigation without being extremely cumbersome. For this reason, pre-clinical, clinical trial and manufacturing experience for an agent is described as part of an investigator's brochure, essentially a 'bible' containing everything known about an agent at the time of writing.

Further reading

A number of useful online sources exist where you can glean the necessary information to construct a clinical trial protocol. Usually your institution or company will have their own template, which you can download. The web link for a typical one from the University of Pittsburgh is:

    ℗ http://www.o3is.pitt.edu/Documents/INDTemplateClinicalStudyProtocol.doc

Clinical study design

Clinical trials

Directive 2001/20/EC defines a clinical trial as any investigation in human subjects intended to discover or verify the clinical, pharmacological, and/ or other pharmacodynamic effects of one or more investigational medicinal product(s), and/or to identify any adverse reactions to one or more investigational medicinal product(s), and/or to study absorption, distribution, metabolism, and excretion of one or more investigational medicinal product(s), with the object of ascertaining its (their) safety and/or efficacy. High-quality study design is vitally important for a successful outcome and the study design will depend upon the aims, the availability of resources and the regulatory and ethical framework.

Phase 0–IV

Phase 0 (microdose) studies are subpharmacological microdose clinical studies (usually less than 100micrograms dose). These studies can evaluate pharmacokinetic (PK) and pharmacodynamic (PD) parameters early in the clinical development programme by employing ultra-sensitive analytic methods. Phase I (pharmacology) studies are small and designed to examine the biological and pharmacological actions, tolerability (maximum tolerated dose), and safety of a new treatment in healthy volunteers or patients. Larger numbers of subjects are recruited to phase II (exploratory) studies and the objective is to define the spectrum of activity (PD, PK) of a new agent administered at an optimal schedule and dose (dose–response relationship). Normally, the study will restrict inclusion criteria to specific patient groups, in line with the known mechanism of action of the active substance. Phase III (confirmatory) trials seek to confirm the activity of the product in a claimed indication, and are designed to substantiate the efficacy and safety profile of the drug. Phase III studies tend to be large (100s–1000s of patients), multinational, multi-centre trials that randomize patients to the test medicinal product vs. a standard of care therapy and/ or placebo. Phase IV (therapeutic use) studies are post-marketing studies, which are important for gathering additional safety data and monitoring efficacy in the patient population.

Clinical trial design

The trial design depends upon the research question that is being asked and key design features include:
• Aim of study (clinical development programme, marketing authorization, investigation of specific properties of a medicinal product, health policy evaluation).
• Type of study question (superiority, equivalence, non-inferiority):
  • Superiority trials aim to show one treatment is superior to another;
  • Equivalence trials aim to show two treatments are not different in a defined way, using pre-determined specific margins.

- Non-inferiority trials aim to show that a new treatment is not worse than a comparator by more than a pre-specified amount, known as the non-inferiority margin or delta.
- Regulatory guidance (ICH, CHMP, GCP), ethics, and scientific advice.
- Study configuration (parallel group, cross-over, factorial).
- Number of centres and recruitment.
- Selection of study population (sample size, inclusion, exclusion criteria).
- Special populations (paediatrics, elderly, hepatic/renal impairment).
- Randomization and method of assignment to treatments, blinding (open, double-blind, single-blind).
- Prior and concomitant therapy.
- Control/comparator arm (placebo, active drug, no treatment, best supportive care, physicians choice, historical).
- Selection and identification of treatments (specific drugs, doses).
- Sequence and duration of study periods.
- Data monitoring or special steering or evaluation committees.
- Statistical analysis plan and interim analysis.
- Definition of outcome measures and efficacy variables (primary and secondary, pharmacology variables).
- Safety evaluation and risk minimization (un/predictable events).
- Pharmaco-economic assessment.
- Biomarker evaluation and validation.

Endpoints and comparator arm

During the clinical development of a novel medicinal product, the definition of clinical benefit is often a challenge and the selected primary endpoint should provide a valid and reliable measure of efficacy in the patient population included in the trial. Endpoints should be selected on the basis of which outcome most accurately reflects the benefit of a new treatment.

The use of a comparison group or control is essential when designing a confirmatory study for regulatory submission and for interpreting research findings. Without a control treatment it is difficult to determine whether a response is due to the effect of the treatment or some other factor. The choice of the comparative intervention depends on the availability of alternative treatments. Control groups may be placebo, best supportive care, no treatment or active treatment. It is generally unethical to give a placebo when an established proven treatment exists because this deprives study subjects of a known health benefit.

- A placebo is an inert preparation, which helps distinguish the pharmacodynamic effects of a drug from the psychological effects of taking a medicine.
- An active treatment is usually the medicine that is most widely prescribed in clinical practice and evidence based where possible.

Further reading

ICH. (1997). General considerations for clinical trials. Available at: ℂ E8http://www.ich.org/filead-min/Public_Web_Site/ICH_Products/Guidelines/Efficacy/E8/Step4/E8_Guideline.pdf

Adaptive trial designs

Overview

Adaptive trial designs allow for alteration to a clinical trial protocol in response to emerging data. The principle is that if it becomes apparent that dosing arms of an in progress phase II programme will not contribute to clinical development, they can be adapted, e.g. by discontinuing ineffective doses or adding new ones as a PK/PD rationale emerges to support their use.

Phase I studies are largely already adaptive; phase II studies are the major place where adaptive trial design may save unnecessary patient exposure to ineffective dose regimens, and consequent time and money.

The Bayesian approach

Bayesian statistics are a key component of the design of adaptive clinical trials. They allow for use of an 'informative prior', where prior experience with a particular agent can be used to modify beliefs around the success of that agent in a particular clinical study.

The advantage is that a rolling probability of success can be calculated either for a trial as a whole, or for individual study arms, thus allowing for discontinuation.

Considerations in adaptive design

A number of surrogates may be useful in adaptive design; examples include glucose, lipid changes, and blood pressure in cardiovascular studies.

Adaptive design and Bayesian statistics may also have a role in rare disease trials, and in paediatric trial design, where there may be very valid reasons for limiting study size due both to recruitment difficulties and expediency of delivery of results.

Some concerns exist around so called seamless phase II/III designs, namely around dose selection, possible bias, and how this can be eliminated by an independent data monitoring committee, and minimizing Type 1 error, Examples do exist, however, of successful adaptive design, specifically in the field of Type 2 diabetes studies.

Future developments

Bayesian statistics and adaptive trial design have become established in phase II clinical trials. Yet to be established is a robust way to develop a seamless transition from phase IIb to phase III. Whilst independent data and safety monitoring committees go some way to allaying fears about this type of study design, many companies would prefer to retain control of the decisions on dosing and engage on further regulatory feedback before progression to studies on clinical efficacy.

Further reading

EMA/EFPIA. EMA/EFPIA 2nd workshop. Adaptive design in confirmatory trials. Available at: ℘ http://www.emea.europa.eu/docs/en_GB/document_library/Minutes/2010/04/WC500089206.pdf

Informed consent

Overview

Informed consent is a decision to participate in research that is taken by a competent individual who has received the necessary information, has adequately understood the information and who, after considering the information, has arrived at a decision without having been subjected to coercion, undue influence or inducement, or intimidation.

Informed consent protects the individual's freedom of choice and respects the individual's autonomy. As an additional safeguard, it must always be complemented by independent ethical review of research proposals. This safeguard of independent review is particularly important as many individuals are limited in their capacity to give adequate informed consent; they include young children, adults with severe mental or behavioural disorders, and persons who are unfamiliar with medical concepts and technology.

The CIOMS guidelines

The CIOMS guidelines state that informed or valid consent must address three questions:
- Does the patient have the capacity to consent requiring consideration of such issues as age, maturity, cognitive ability?
- Is the consent voluntary (i.e. is the decision made free from coercion, inducement, or intimidation including pressure from a family member)?
- Has the patient received sufficient information on which to base his/her decision?

Patients need to have time to study information and ask additional questions before being asked to make a decision. Information should be available in appropriate languages and written in a style that is understandable by patients, taking into consideration relevant factors, including cultural differences. In addition, the CIOMS guidelines stipulate that the consent process must be documented, and the use of biologic materials, including their possible storage and future use and whether the material will be anonymized, needs to be frankly discussed. Finally, the CIOMS guidelines recommend the use of a checklist to guide the consenting process (see Box 4.6.1).

In obtaining and documenting informed consent, the investigator should comply with the applicable regulatory requirement(s), and should adhere to GCP and to the ethical principles that have their origin in the Declaration of Helsinki.

Box 4.6.1 The CIOMS guidelines

- Inform the subject why they are being approached.
- Ensure that consent in voluntary.
- Explain freedom to withdraw.
- Explain the purpose of the research.
- Describe the trial design in lay terms.
- Explain duration of participation required.
- Discuss any remuneration.
- Discuss mechanisms to inform participants of study results.
- Notify participant of confidentiality arrangements and safeguards about access to data.
- Confirm ethical review has been obtained.
- Discuss foreseeable risks.
- Discuss possible benefits to the individual or community.
- Will the treatment be available after study completion?
- What are the alternative treatments to study medication or therapy?
- Are any secondary studies proposed?
- Is there a distinction between the role of the investigator and the patient's physician?
- Are medical services provided for the subject during the study?
- Explain what arrangements have been made to deal with research-related injury.
- How will the subject be compensated in the event of research-related injury?

Reproduced with permission from the *International Ethical Guidelines for Biomedical Research Involving Human Subjects*: Prepared by the Council for International Organizations of Medical Sciences (CIOMS) in collaboration with the World Health Organization (WHO), copyright CIOMS, Geneva 2002.

Further reading

International Ethical Guidelines for Biomedical Research Involving Human Subjects: Prepared by the Council for International Organizations of Medical Sciences (CIOMS) in collaboration with the World Health Organization (WHO). Geneva: CIOMS, 2002.

The Council for International Organizations and Medical Sciences (CIOMS). Guidelines on Ethics of Clinical Trials. *Proc Am Thorac Soc*, 2007; 4: 176–9.

ICH Topic E6 (R1). Guideline for good clinical practice. July 2002. Available at: ℅ http://www.edctp.org/fileadmin/documents/EMEA_ICH-GCP_Guidelines_July_2002

Chapter 4.7

Data protection

Overview

The Data Protection Act 1998 commenced on 1 March 2000, with most of its provisions being effective from 24 October 2001. The purpose of the Act is to protect the rights and privacy of individuals, and to ensure that data about them are not processed without their knowledge and are processed with their consent wherever possible.

The eight principles

The Data Protection Act of 1998 states that anyone processing personal data must comply with the eight enforceable principles of good practice, as shown in Box 4.7.1.

Box 4.7.1 The eight principles of the Data Protection Act

Data must be:
- Fairly and lawfully processed.
- Processed for limited purposes.
- Adequate, relevant and not excessive.
- Accurate.
- Not kept longer than necessary.
- Processed in accordance with the data subject's rights.
- Secure.
- Not transferred to countries without adequate protection.

Those involved in clinical research should be aware the processing of any information relating to an identifiable living individual constitutes 'personal data processing' and is therefore subject to the provisions of the 1998 Act, including the eight data protection principles set out in Box 4.7.1.

Research exemption

However, there are certain exemptions in the 1998 Act relating to the processing of data for research. These are defined by Section 33, and relate to principles 2, 5, and 7, and to Section 7. These exemptions apply only where:
- The data are *not* processed to support measures or decisions with respect to particular individuals.
- The processing of data for research will *not* cause substantial damage and distress to any data subject.

For the exemptions to apply, the research activity must fulfil *all* of the following conditions:
- The personal data is being used exclusively for research purposes (includes statistical or historical research purposes).

- The personal data must have no other use, not even incidental use.
- The personal data is not being used to support measures or decisions relating to any identifiable living individual (not just the data subject but anyone who may be affected by your research).
- The personal data is not being used in a way that will cause, or is likely to cause, substantial damage or substantial distress to any data subject.
- The results of the research activity, or any resulting statistics, must not be available in a form that identifies the data subjects, e.g. the use of case studies in a research report and disguising the names of the individuals. However, if their circumstances are described in detail it may be possible for someone to identify that individual.

It is important that researchers remember that there are *no* blanket exemptions from the data protection principles set out in Box 4.7.1. It is important that those undertaking research, both staff or students, are aware that most of the data protection principles still apply. They need to be aware of where and when they apply.

Further reading

Data Protection Act 1998. Available at: ✍ http://www.legislation.org.uk/

Indemnity and compensation

Overview

Model agreements governing indemnity and compensation for institutions and individuals taking part in industry-sponsored clinical trials exist across all countries where studies are run.

These all incorporate standard elements:

- All elements of the study have to be individually approvable, i.e. protocol, investigator's brochure (IB), informed consent, ethics board review, etc.
- Financial arrangements should be acceptable.
- Negligence is not covered under any indemnity agreement.

Compensation and liability

- In general, sponsors will be liable for adverse events due to innate properties of the trial drug or effects of procedures associated with the conduct of the trial, whereas liability due to errors in the formulation, dilution, or administration of the drug or errors in conduct of the trial will fall on the parties that erred.
- In the USA, there are no national regulations requiring sponsors and institutions to provide free medical care or compensation for injuries due to clinical trials, but some institutions have specific policies on compensation.
- In Europe, the 2001 European Directive on the conduct of clinical trials requires that provision be made for insurance or indemnity to cover the liability of the investigator and the sponsor before a trial can be undertaken.
- Any company carrying out studies makes provision for insurance that will cover them against possible claims. Investigators are advised to check their personal medical indemnity cover to ensure they are covered for participation in clinical trials as an investigator.

Level of payment made

In general, guidelines suggest that the level of payment made should be appropriate to the nature, severity, and persistence of the injury, and be in line with compensation paid in a court of local jurisdiction.

The amount paid may be ameliorated according to the seriousness of any disease being treated in a phase II or III clinical study, the probability of adverse reactions occurring, and any warnings that have been provided.

It may also be ameliorated according to the risks and benefits of pre-existing treatments for the disease.

Further reading

ABPI. Model indemnity agreement. Available at: ℘ http://www.abpi.org.uk/our-work/library/guide-lines/Pages/indemnity-england-wales.aspx
Steinbrook R (2006). Compensation for injured research subjects. *N Engl J Med* **354**(18), 1871–3.

ABPI. Clinical trial compensation guidelines, 1994. Available at: 🔗 http://www.abpi.org.uk/our-work/library/guidelines/Pages/ct-compensation.aspx

Landing site for MDU commentary on involvement in clinical research. Available at: 🔗 http://www.the-mdu.com/section_medical_students/topnav_news_3/hidden_article.asp?articleid=2168&contenttype=media+release&articletitle=be+aware+of+research+risks+advises+mdu

Chapter 4.9

Investigator's brochure

Overview

The IB is a compilation of the clinical and non-clinical data on the investigational product(s) that are relevant to the study of the product(s) in human subjects.

Its purpose is to provide the investigators and others involved in the trial with the information to facilitate their understanding of the rationale for, and their compliance with, many key features of the protocol, such as:

• The dose.
• Dose frequency/interval.
• Methods of administration.
• Safety monitoring procedures.

The IB also provides insight to support the clinical management of the study subjects during the course of the clinical trial. The information should be presented in a concise, simple, objective, balanced, and non-promotional form that enables a clinician or potential investigator to understand it and make his/her own unbiased risk–benefit assessment of the appropriateness of the proposed trial. For this reason, a medically qualified person should generally participate in the editing of an IB, but the contents of the IB should be approved by the disciplines that generated the described data.

Minimum information required

The ICH Topic E6(R1), Guideline for good clinical practice, delineates the minimum information that should be included in an IB and provides suggestions for its layout (see Box 4.9.1).

Box 4.9.1 Table of contents of investigator's brochure

• Confidentiality statement (optional).
• Signature page (optional).
  1. Table of contents.
  2. Summary.
  3. Introduction.
  4. Physical, chemical, and pharmaceutical properties, and formulation.
     Non-clinical studies
  5.1 Non-clinical pharmacology.
  5.2 Pharmacokinetics and product metabolism in animals.
     Effects in humans.
  6.1 Pharmacokinetics and product metabolism in humans.
  6.2 Safety and efficacy.
  6.3 Marketing experience.
     Summary of data and guidance for the investigator.

The type and extent of information available will vary with the stage of development of the investigational product. If the investigational product is marketed and its pharmacology is widely understood by medical practitioners, an extensive IB may not be necessary. Where permitted by regulatory authorities, a basic product information brochure, package leaflet, or labelling may be an appropriate alternative, provided that it includes current, comprehensive, and detailed information on all aspects of the investigational product that might be of importance to the investigator.

Review period

The IB should be reviewed at least annually and revised as necessary in compliance with a sponsor's written procedures. More frequent revision may be appropriate depending on the stage of development and the generation of relevant new information.

However, in accordance with Good Clinical Practice, relevant new information may be so important that it should be communicated to the investigators, and possibly to the IRBs/IECs, and/or regulatory authorities before it is included in a revised IB.

Generally, the sponsor is responsible for ensuring that an up-to-date IB is made available to the investigator(s), and the investigators are responsible for providing the up-to-date IB to the responsible IRBs/IECs. In the case of an investigator sponsored trial, the sponsor–investigator should determine whether a brochure is available from the commercial manufacturer. If the investigational product is provided by the sponsor–investigator, then he or she should provide the necessary information to the trial personnel. In cases where preparation of a formal IB is impractical, the sponsor–investigator should provide, as a substitute, an expanded background information section in the trial protocol that contains the minimum current information described in this guideline.

Further reading

ICH Topic E6(R1). Guideline for good clinical practice. CPMP/ICH/135/95. Available at: ⅍ http://www.emea.europa.eu/docs/en_GB/document_library/Scientific_guideline/2009/09/ WC500002874.pdf

Organization of project teams/project planning

Overview

A number of essential team members are defined with respect to effective operation of clinical project teams, and what their roles entail. Project management training is also available for physician team members.

Essential team members

Project manager

Defines the project scope, lifecycle, constraints, risk assessment; agrees responsibilities, work plan, critical path analysis, tracks and deals with variance from the plan, essentially the glue that sticks everyone together and keeps everyone on track.

Physician

Assesses applicability of trial endpoints for registration and reimbursement, feasibility of trial, dealing with external agencies, investigators, training, medical monitoring.

Regulatory

Assessment of manufacturing, pre-clinical and clinical package required for registration. Regulatory responsibility may often be split between a CMC expert and an expert on the clinical package.

CMC/clinical trial supplies/manufacturing

Delivering stability package necessary to conduct studies and for commercial production. Also responsible for logistics of making medication strengths/placebo/comparator medication available for studies.

Pre-clinical scientist

Delivering the package of pre-clinical/animal data required to conduct late phase clinical trials and for registration. This includes data such as carcinogenicity assessment and reproductive toxicity assessment where appropriate.

Key features that should be contained in a clinical trial project plan

- Identify and allocate resourcing for the clinical trial plan and set up timelines for the project.
- How to manage resourcing during the trial itself.
- Budget including phased spend.
- Identify which stakeholders need to review the project and how can the team work most effectively with them.
- Identify risk and strategies to mitigate potential risks.
- Plan to actively control the progress of the study.
- Strategies to identify and manage issues as they arise.

Further reading

Association for Project Management. Available at: ◌ http://www.apm.org.uk/

Clinical trial project management course link:

◌ http://www.lshtm.ac.uk/prospectus/short/dlmodules/ctm203.pdf

Chapter 4.11

Contractual arrangements with research sites and contract research organizations

Overview

Pharmaceutical, biotech, and other research-based organizations ('sponsors') who act as study sponsors, often run studies in-house, but there is a trend towards increased outsourcing of this activity to clinical research organizations (CRO). Contractual arrangements must be in place for either eventuality. However, a different agreement is required depending on whether the contract is with the study site or the CRO. Therefore, clinical trial agreements (CTAgs) are used to contract with research sites to conduct clinical trials and service agreements (SAs) are used to contract with CROs.

While there are similarities between the two types of contracts, they reflect the different relationship that the sponsor has with both the research site and the CRO.

The difference between the contracts stems from 2 areas.
- Agreement with CRO is based on buying services, while agreement with a research site is based on acquiring data.
- The scale of the agreements are far greater in the case of service agreements so significant negotiation can be expected.

Agreement comparison

The differences between the agreements can be captured in considering the areas in Box 4.11.1.

Box 4.11.1 Areas of comparison
- Delegation of authority.
- Intellectual property **and** publication rights.
- Study staff.
- Liability insurance.
- SOPs.
- Changes to service or study.
- Delays.

Delegation of authority
Within a service agreement, it is necessary for the sponsor to delegate some authority to the CRO. However, within a CTAgs, the sponsor does not delegate authority.

Intellectual property and publication rights
In an SA, the CRO does not have any intellectual property or publication rights. These are retained by the sponsor. However, there may be some instances within a CTAgs when the site will have publication rights and rights of data ownership.

Study staff

The sponsor can dictate the staffing levels required by the CRO in managing the study and can also dictate the assignment of key staff as required. In a CTAgs, the study site is chosen based on the existing resource and minimum acceptable criteria. However, it may terminate the agreement if the principal investigator leaves the study without an acceptable replacement.

Liability insurance

While a CRO must have professional liability insurance, the site is only required to have medical malpractice insurance.

Standard operating procedures

In an SA, the sponsor may either review the CRO's SOPs to assess their acceptability or they may require that the CRO uses the sponsors own SOPs. It is not required that the site follow the sponsors SOP, but they must adhere to the study protocol.

Changes to service or study

Any changes to the study may require additional payment. This is not generally the case in CTAgs.

Study delays

The sponsor must reimburse the CRO for any study delays. This is not usual in the case of a CTAgs.

Case report form

Case report form

All clinical trials require a mechanism for formally documenting the characteristics and parameters of study subjects, from the point of study entry to trial exit. The case report form (CRF) is the official data recording document used during a clinical trial. Data gathered from CRFs enables the generation of a variety of study reports and analyses.

The design and completeness of a CRF directly affects the success or failure of a clinical trial. The CRF must be designed well in advance of a clinical study and should adequately capture and record data for each subject. Data collected from trial subjects may come from clinical records, assessments, tests, or questionnaires. These data are used to evaluate pharmacology, efficacy, and safety, and ultimately fulfil the trial objectives. The clinical trial protocol determines what data should be collected in the CRF and this may include the following elements:

- Eligibility checklist.
- Patient identification.
- Disease history.
- Previous treatment.
- Physical examination and assessment of pre-existing disease.
- Routine laboratory measurements.
- Research procedures.
- Allocated intervention.
- Permitted concomitant treatments.
- Variables to measure treatment effect.
- Adverse events and other safety considerations.

Ideally, the CRF should be simple and quick to complete, and should be developed by a multidisciplinary team. The investigators and other study personnel should have an opportunity to review the CRF during the developmental stage in order to ensure that all the important information will be captured and the text is unambiguous in nature. CRFs should be designed to collect data required by the study protocol and no more and a well-designed CRF facilitates data collection and entry. Over-ambitious attempts to include too many variables may result in complex forms that are impractical and difficult to use.

Trial personnel should be trained to efficiently complete and fully capture the information required for the CRFs. The CRF may be either in a printed paper or an electronic format, and increasingly data is entered electronically in a trial data base such as an electronic data capture (EDC) system. EDC has several advantages over paper, including reducing the chances of error, eliminating duplication of repetitive data, and facilitating data analysis. Currently, there are a number of initiatives that attempt to standardize CRFs by establishing core libraries of harmonized and standardized phase II and phase III CRFs. The following points should be considered when designing a CRF:

- Only collect relevant data in accordance with the trial protocol and in compliance with regulatory requirements.
- Collect data which allows for computerization and facilitates data analysis.

- Involve team members at all stages of development of the CRF.
- Include organized, clear, and concise modules that promote accurate data collection.
- Avoid duplication and ambiguous statements.
- Actual numbers and values should be documented, rather than calculated values.
- Provide standard units or references ranges.
- Design minimal free text responses wherever possible.
- Include instructions for use in order to reduce misinterpretation.
- Include a header and footer with study number, centre, and subject identification number.

Good clinical practice and the case report form

The content of a CRF should reflect the source documents, such as medical records, pharmacy notes, and questionnaires. It is important that any information recorded on CRFs can be independently verified for audit purposes or for GCP inspections. According to ICH Topic E6, Guideline for good clinical practice:

- The investigator should ensure the accuracy, completeness, legibility, and timeliness of the data reported to the sponsor in the CRFs.
- Data reported on the CRF, that are derived from source documents, should be consistent with the source documents or the discrepancies should be explained.
- Any change or correction to a CRF should be dated, initialled, and explained, and should not obscure the original entry (i.e. an audit trail should be maintained).

Further reading

ICH. Guideline for good clinical practice E6(R1). Available at: ℘ http://www.ich.org/fileadmin/Public_Web_Site/ICH_Products/Guidelines/Efficacy/E6_R1/Step4/E6_R1__Guideline.pdf

ICH. Efficacy guidelines. Available at: ℘ http://www.ich.org/products/guidelines/efficacy/article/efficacy-guidelines.html

Chapter 4.13

Budgeting and cost control

Factors that impact clinical trial costs

A number of factors can impact clinical trial costs, and should be taken into account when budgeting for a study. These include:
- Therapeutic area.
- Phase of development.
- Country.
- Advertising.
- Time.
- Electronic data capture.
- Use of CRO.

Any or all of these factors can significantly impact on study budgeting, with ophthalmology studies traditionally very cheap, on a per-patient cost basis, vs. psychiatry studies, which have traditionally been very expensive. Invasive and more frequent monitoring, a necessity in early phase studies, also impacts significantly on study costs.

Building a clinical trial budget

External costs
- Subject fees (grants).
- CRO costs.
- Drug costs.
- Other costs, e.g.:
  - Investigator meeting.
  - Printing.
  - Equipment.
  - Interactive voice recognition system (IVRS).
  - CRF.
  - Central laboratory.
  - Central electrocardiogram (ECG).
  - Steering committee.
  - Data Safety Monitoring Board (DSMB), etc.

Internal costs
- Fixed costs (e.g. buildings and headcount).
- Operational costs.

Feasibility/benchmarking

Feasibility and benchmarking are crucial with respect to cost control. Benchmark costs exist by country for the range of standard clinical trial investigations, and hospital and general practice consultations. Benchmark costs should always be compared against those collected as part of feasibility, and it's important to remember that key experts may well not be the best recruiters from a trial point of view.

Internal activity
See Table 4.13.1.

Custom budget for each country: factors that can impact on differences between in-country costs
- Procedure costs.
- IRB or ethics committee fees.
- Legal issues.
- Subject compensation.
- Advertising practices.
- Incentive payment.
- Equipment costs.
- Central laboratory use.
- Regularly review progress against metrics, allows for remedial action to be taken.
- Stage payments, always more incentive for trialists to perform when payments are made according to milestone review.
- Use finance support to review costs against predicted spend.

Table 4.13.1 Average work capacity per staff member

CRA can monitor	10–15 sites
MD/PhD can manage	50–75 sites
1.5–2.0 data technician can support	1 statistician
1 programmer can support	5–10 reports/yr
1 statistician can analyse	5–10 studies/yr
Medical writer can prepare	4–6 reports/yr

Expanded access programmes

Overview

Expanded access programmes are a way of making a promising medicine available to patients with significant unmet need, before it has actually gained marketing authorization. Both FDA and EMA have very specific guidelines on the setting up and administration of expanded access programmes.

Which diseases qualify?

Only diseases that are serious, life-threatening, long-lasting, or significantly disabling can qualify for an expanded access programme. Examples may include rare cancers for which existing therapies are limited, or serious genetic disorders such as muscular dystrophy for instance.

In essence, it must be established that the risk from the drug is unlikely to be greater than the risk from the disease, based on the evidence so far obtained.

What are the nuts and bolts of expanded access for the company concerned?

Manufacturers are not always willing and able to provide expanded access programmes for investigational drugs. Under the FDA rules they are allowed to charge for the agent if covering a cost for provision is required, and any access programme has to be under the control of an IRB. Similar rules are in place for the EU, where each country competent authority where a drug is made available for compassionate use must keep a register.

Does the EMA recommend which investigational agents can qualify for compassionate use?

Yes it does.

The EMAs Committee for Medicinal Products for Human Use (CHMP) can provide recommendations to all EU MSs on how to administer, distribute, and use certain medicines for compassionate use. It does also identify which patients may benefit from compassionate use programmes.

The Committee can provide these recommendations at the request of a MS. It can also do so when it becomes aware that compassionate use programmes with a given medicine are being set up in a number of MSs.

What are some of the advantages and drawbacks of expanded use programmes?

The major advantage is that after an efficacy trial has reported, patients with significant unmet needs have the opportunity to benefit from a medicine with proven efficacy, whilst it is undergoing the registration process.

A potential disadvantage is that expanded access may limit recruitment to further randomized controlled trials, and unblinded data may be difficult to interpret against other blinded RCT data.

Further reading

EMA. Questions and answers on the compassionate use of medicines in the European Union. Available at: ✏ http://www.ema.europa.eu/docs/en_GB/document_library/Other/2010/01/WC 500069898.pdf

✏ http://edocket.access.gpo.gov/2009/pdf/E9–19005.pdf

Study master file preparation

Before the clinical phase of the trial commences

During this planning stage, the following documents should be generated and should be on file before the trial formally starts:

- *Investigator's brochure:*
  - To document that relevant and current scientific information about the investigational product has been provided to the investigator.
  - File of the investigator and sponsor.
- *Signed protocol and amendments, if any, and sample case report form:*
  - To document investigator and sponsor agreement to the protocol/ amendment(s) and case report form.
  - File of the investigator and sponsor.
- *Information given to trial subjects: Informed consent form (including all applicable translations):*
  - To document the informed consent.
  - File of the investigator and sponsor.
- *Information given to trial subjects and any other written information:*
  - To document that subjects will be given appropriate written information (content and wording) to support their ability to give fully informed consent.
  - File of the investigator and sponsor.
- *Information given to trial subjects and advertisement for subject recruitment (if used):*
  - To document that recruitment measures are appropriate and not coercive.
  - File of the investigator.
- *Financial aspects of the trial:*
  - To document the financial agreement between the investigator/ institution and the sponsor for the trial.
  - File of the investigator and sponsor.
- *Insurance statement (where required):*
  - To document that compensation to subject(s) for trial-related injury will be available.
  - File of the investigator and sponsor.
- *Signed agreement between involved parties:* file of the investigator and sponsor.
- *Dated, documented favourable opinion of Ethics Committee on the full range of study documentation, compensation, etc.:* file of the investigator and sponsor.
- *Ethics Committee composition:*
  - To document that the Ethics Committee is constituted in agreement with GCP.
  - File of the investigator and sponsor (where required).
- *Regulatory authority(ies) authorization/approval/notification of protocol:*
  - To document appropriate authorization/approval/notification by the regulatory authority(ies) has been obtained prior to initiation of the trial in compliance with the applicable regulatory requirement(s).

- • File of the investigator and sponsor (where required).
- • *Curriculum vitae and/or other relevant documents evidencing qualifications of investigator(s) and/or supporting trial staff to whom investigator tasks are delegated:*
  - • To document qualifications and eligibility to conduct trial and/or provide medical supervision.
  - • File of the investigator and sponsor (where required).
- • *Normal value(s)/range(s) for medical/laboratory/technical procedure(s) and/or test(s) included in the protocol:* file of the investigator and sponsor.
- • *Medical/laboratory/technical procedures/tests:* file of the investigator (where required) and sponsor.
- • *Sample of label(s) attached to investigational medicinal product container(s):* file of the sponsor.
- • *Instructions for handling of investigational medicinal product(s) and trial related materials:*
  - • (If not included in protocol or IB).
  - • File of the investigator and sponsor.
- • *Distribution records for investigational medicinal product(s) and trial related materials:* file of the investigator and sponsor.
- • *Certificate(s) of analysis of investigational product(s):* file of the sponsor and investigator.
- • *Decoding procedures for blinded trials:* file of the investigator and sponsor (third party if applicable).
- • *Master randomization list:* file of the sponsor (third party if applicable).
- • *Pre-trial monitoring report:* file of the sponsor.
- • *Trial initiation monitoring report:* file of the investigator and sponsor.

During the clinical conduct of the trial

In addition to having on file the documents (see 'Before the clinical phase of the trial commences', p. 243), the following should be added to the files during the trial as evidence that all new relevant information is documented as it becomes available.

- • *Investigator's brochure updates:* file of the investigator and sponsor.
- • *Any revision to:*
  - • Protocol/amendment(s) and case report form.
  - • Informed consent form.
  - • Any other written information provided to subjects.
  - • Advertisement for subject recruitment (if used).
  - • File of the investigator and sponsor.
- • *Dated, documented favourable opinion of the Ethics Committee on any revision to the study or materials:* file of the investigator and sponsor.
- • *Regulatory authority(ies) authorizations/approvals/notifications where required for any revisions to the study or materials:* file of the investigator (where required) and sponsor.
- • *Curriculum vitae for new investigator(s) and/or supporting trial staff to whom investigator tasks are delegated:* file of the investigator and sponsor.

- *Updates to normal value(s)/range(s) for medical/laboratory/ technical procedure(s)/test(s) included in the protocol:* file of the investigator and sponsor.
- *Updates of medical/laboratory/technical procedures/tests:* file of the investigator (where required) and sponsor.
- *Documentation of investigational medicinal product(s) and trial related materials distribution:* file of the investigator and sponsor.
- *Certificate(s) of analysis for new batches of investigational products:* file of the sponsor.
- *Monitoring visit reports:* file of the sponsor.
- *Relevant communications other than site visits:* file of the investigator and sponsor.
- *Signed informed consent forms:* file of the investigator.
- *Source documents:* file of the investigator.
- *Signed, dated, and completed case report forms:* file of the investigator (copy) and sponsor (original).
- *Documentation of case report form corrections:* file of the investigator(copy) and sponsor (original).

- *Notification by originating investigator to sponsor of serious adverse events and related reports:* file of the investigator and sponsor.
- *Notification by sponsor and/or investigator, where applicable, to regulatory authority(ies) and Ethics Committees of suspected unexpected serious adverse reactions and of other safety information:* file of the investigator (where required) and sponsor.
- *Notification by sponsor to investigators of safety information in accordance with 'The detailed guidance on the collection, verification and presentation of adverse reaction reports arising from clinical trials on medicinal products for human use':* file of the investigator and sponsor.
- Interim or annual reports to Ethics Committees and authority(ies).
- *Interim or annual reports provided to Ethics Committees and to authorities:* file of the investigator and sponsor (where required).
- *Subject screening log:* file of the investigator and sponsor (where required).
- *Subject identification code list:* file of the investigator.
- *Subject enrolment log:* file of the investigator.
- *Investigational medicinal product accountability at the site:* file of the investigator and sponsor.
- *Signature sheet:*
  - To document signatures and initials of all persons authorized to make entries and/or corrections on case report forms.
  - File of the investigator and sponsor.
- *Record of retained body fluids/tissue samples (if any):* file of the investigator and sponsor.

After completion or termination of the trial

After completion or termination of the trial, all of the documents identified (see 'Before the clinical phase of the trial commences', p. 243, and 'During the clinical conduct of the trial', p. 244) should be in the file together with the following:

- *Investigational medicinal product(s) accountability at site:* file of the investigator and sponsor.
- *Documentation of investigational product destruction:* file of the investigator (if destroyed at site) and sponsor.
- *Completed subject identification code list:* file of the investigator.
- *Audit certificate:* file of the sponsor.
- *Final trial close-out monitoring report:* file of the sponsor.
- *Treatment allocation and decoding documentation:* file of the sponsor.
- *Final report by investigator to Ethics Committees where required, and, where applicable, to the regulatory authority(ies):* file of the investigator.
- *Clinical study report:* file of the investigator (if applicable) and sponsor.

Quality of essential documents

Essential documents should be complete, legible, accurate, and unambiguous. They should be signed and dated as appropriate.

Media to be used

Directive 2005/28/EC states in Article 20 that: 'The media used to store essential documents shall be such that those documents remain complete and legible throughout the required period of retention and can be made available to the competent authorities upon request. Any alteration to records shall be traceable.'[1]

[1] Reproduced with permission from 'Commission Directive 2005/28/EC of 8 April 2005 laying down principles and detailed guidelines for good clinical practice as regards investigational medicinal products for human use, as well as the requirements for authorisation of the manufacturing or importation of such products', OJ L 91, 9.4.2005, ✎ http://eur-lex.europa.eu, © European Union, 1998–2012.

Further reading

Europa (2006). Recommendation on the content of the trial master file and archiving. Available at: ✎ http://ec.europa.eu/health/files/eudralex/vol-10/v10_chap5_en.pdf

Target product profile

Overview

The target product profile (TPP) essentially acts as a 1-page road map to guide clinical development. In its original form, the TPP was intended to act as a road map for clinical development to develop a particular label. As industry has realized, the need to provide data that is appropriate for clinical context and reimbursement, the TPP has metamorphosed over the past few years into a target market profile or TMP, which incorporates not only the clinical plan needed to deliver a particular label, but also that needed to deliver data in a segment appropriate for reimbursement.

What does the target product profile consist of?

Ideally, the TPP should consist of the answers to 3 main questions:
• What is the major unmet need in the population you are targeting your drug at?
• What are the major attributes for your particular drug that will meet those needs?
• How will you demonstrate those needs in your clinical trial programme?

An example could come from the world of Type 2 diabetes:

What is the major unmet need in the population you are targeting your drug for?
Answer Long-term glycaemic control with a safety profile similar to the dipeptidyl peptidase IV (DPPIV) inhibitors (no hypoglycaemia, significant adverse effects), with demonstrated cardiovascular benefit.

What are the major attributes for your particular drug which will meet those needs?
Answer HbA1c reductions at least as effective as the leading branded agent on the market, safety profile like the DPPIV inhibitors, reduction in major adverse cardiovascular endpoints (MACE).

How will you demonstrate those needs in your clinical trial programme?
Answer A list of proposed trials, e.g. 6-month add-in to standard blood glucose lowering treatment vs. branded comparator, 3-year curriculum vitae (CV) study looking at MACE endpoints, glucose monitoring to look for hypoglycaemia, etc.

How does the regulator see the target product profile?

TPPs are not compulsory, and may submitted as part of the end of phase 2 FDA review process on a voluntary basis. What the FDA look for is slightly different with respect to the TPP, and they have given specific guidance; the web link for this is provided in Further reading.

How does the industry use the target product profile?

The major use in industry is as a road map, which details important activities with respect to the clinical trial programme, and helps sequence the timing of when these should be put in place. It also serves to set criteria, particularly when unmet needs or major attributes for a particular drug are considered, with respect to go/no-go decisions.

A drug that is intended for Type 2 diabetes, for example, is likely to cease development if it shows an adverse signal with respect to cholesterol during the phase 2a programme.

TPPs for the 'ideal' drug in a particular indication are also created to guide early phase pipeline groups and business development groups within big pharma. There may be early mechanistic hints that a particular drug will satisfy an unmet need, and another rival pharma group may have an agent that fits your TPP, driving a willingness for negotiations about partnering.

How often should the target product profile be revisited?

The TPP is a living document, it isn't set in stone from the first moment a drug leaves the pre-clinical trial world and enters phase 1. It's crucial to revisit the TPP at each stage after clinical trial information becomes available from phase 1 to phase 3, to determine whether it accurately reflects all available information.

Further reading

FDA. Guidance for industry and review staff target product profile—a strategic development process tool. Available at: ℘ http://www.fda.gov/downloads/Drugs/GuidanceComplianceRegulatory Information/Guidances/ucm080593.pdf

Tebbey PW, Rink C (2009). Target product profile: a renaissance for its definition and use. J Med Mark **9**(4):301–7. Available at: ℘ http://www.imshealth.com/imshealth/Global/Content/ Document/Target_Product_Profile.pdf

Section 5

Statistics and data management

Chapter 5.1

Determining the sample size in a clinical trial

Overview

Sample size determination is an important part of planning for clinical trials. One of the key aspects of the protocol is sample size estimation. The goal is to ensure that a trial is large enough to detect reliably the smallest possible differences in the primary outcome, with treatment that is considered clinically worthwhile. It is possible for studies to be underpowered, failing to detect even large treatment effects because of inadequate sample size.

Therefore, sample size must be planned carefully to ensure that the resources invested including patient participation, are not wasted. It may be considered unethical to recruit patients into a study that does not have a large enough sample size to deliver meaningful information.

Elements of sample size calculation

The minimum information required to calculate the sample size for a randomized controlled trial includes:
• Power.
• The level of significance.
• Underlying event rate in the population under investigation.
• Size of the treatment effect sought.

Power

The power of a study is its ability to detect a true difference in outcome between the control arm and the intervention arm. Sample size increases as power increases. The higher the power, the lower the chance of missing a real effect of treatments. Type II error is directly proportional to sample size.

As per ICH E9 guideline, power should not be less than 80%. A study power set at 80% accepts a likelihood of one in five (that is, 20%) of missing a real difference.

Level of significance

This is an important consideration as the level of significance determines the likelihood of detecting a treatment effect when no effect exists (a 'false-positive' result). It also defines the threshold 'P value.' Results with a P value above the threshold lead to the conclusion that an observed difference may be due to chance alone, while those with a P value below the threshold lead to rejecting the null hypothesis and concluding that the intervention has a real effect. It is most commonly taken as 5% (that is, $P = 0.05$) or 1% ($P = 0.01$). This means the investigator accepts a 5% (or 1%) chance of incorrectly reporting a significant effect.

Underlying population event rate

Great care is required in specifying the event rate. Unlike the statistical power and level of significance, which are generally chosen by convention, the underlying expected event must be established by other means, such as previous studies. If an event rate is low, a larger sample size is required.

Therefore, it is advisable to have allowed for sample size adjustment should the overall event rate prove to be lower than anticipated.

Size of treatment effect

This must take into account that there may be a conflict between the actual effect of treatment and the anticipated effect.

Studies can be designed to identify an anticipated large treatment effect requiring a smaller sample size. However, if the actual effect is lower, while it may well still be important, it will be rendered statistically non-significant as the sample size is too small. Therefore, rather than speculate on large differences, one may wish to use the smallest difference that will be of clinical importance.

CONSORT checklist

CONSORT have provided a checklist for determining the sample size for a clinical trial (see Box 5.1.1).

Box 5.1.1 CONSORT checklist for determining sample size for clinical trials

- Estimate the event rate in the control group by extrapolating from a population similar to the population expected in the trial.
- Determine, for the primary outcome, the smallest difference that will be of clinical importance.
- Determine the clinically justifiable power for the particular trial.
- Determine the significance level or probability of a 'false positive' result that is scientifically acceptable.
- Adjust the calculated sample size for the expected level of non-compliance with treatment.

Reproduced with permission from Altman DG, Schulz KF, Moher D, et al, for the CONSORT group. 'The revised CONSORT statement for reporting randomized trials: explanation and elaboration ', *Ann Intern Med* 2001; **134**: 663–94.

Further reading

Altman DG, Schulz KF, Moher D, et al., for the CONSORT group. The revised CONSORT statement for reporting randomized trials: explanation and elaboration. *Ann Intern Med* 2001; **134**: 663–94.

ICH Topic E9 (1998). Statistical principles for clinical trials. CPMP/ICH/363/96. Available at: ℳ http://www.emea.europa.eu/docs/en_GB/document_library/Scientific_guideline/2009/09/WC500002928.pdf

Sensitivity and specificity

Overview

These two measures are closely related to the concepts of type I and type II errors.

Imagine a study evaluating a new screening test for ovarian cancer. Each person taking the test either has or does not have ovarian cancer. The test results for each subject may or may not match the subject's actual status. In that setting:

- *True positive:* people with ovarian cancer actually have ovarian cancer.
- *False positive:* healthy people incorrectly identified as having ovarian cancer.
- *True negative:* healthy people correctly identified as healthy.
- *False negative:* people with ovarian cancer incorrectly identified as healthy.

Calculating sensitivity and specificity

Sensitivity measures the proportion of actual positives which are correctly identified as such (e.g. the percentage of people with ovarian cancer who are correctly identified as having the condition).

This can be calculated using this equation:

Sensitivity = No. true +ves/(No. true +ves + No. false −ves)

Therefore, if a test has a high sensitivity, a negative result would provide a level of confidence of the absence of disease. If any given test has 100% sensitivity, then all people with the disease will be identified, but some may be identified in error. In order to make a decision on the clinical utility of this test, one must be able to quantify the number of patients who are incorrectly identified. Therefore, the sensitivity alone cannot be used to determine whether a test is useful in practice.

Specificity measures the proportion of negatives which are correctly identified (e.g. the percentage of healthy people who are correctly identified as not having the condition).

Specificity = No. true −ves/(No. true −ves + No. false +ves)

Therefore, a test with a high specificity, a positive test result would suggest that it is highly probable that the disease is indeed present. Similarly, if a test has 100% specificity, while people who do not have the disease will always be correctly identified, some patients will be reassured in error. Therefore, the specificity alone cannot be used to determine whether a test is useful in practice.

Ideally, one aims to achieve 100% sensitivity and 100% specificity. However in reality, there is usually a trade-off between the measures. A test with a high sensitivity has a low type II error rate (see Fig. 5.2.1). A test with a high specificity has a low type I error rate.

A hypothetical worked example is shown in Fig. 5.2.2. An ultrasound screening test for ovarian cancer was used on 1000 women.

Therefore, with a large false positive rate and a low false negative rate suggests that this test was relatively poor at confirming ovarian cancer. However, a negative result is very reassuring as it correctly identified 93% of patients who do not have ovarian cancer.

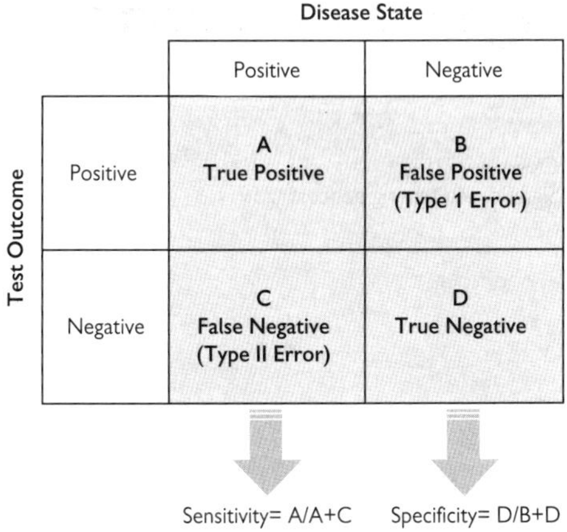

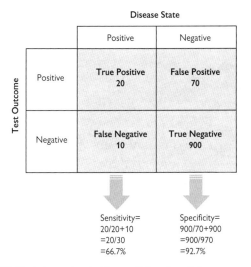

Fig 5.2.1 Calculating sensitivity and specificity.

Fig 5.2.2 Worked example: calculating sensitivity and specificity.

Chapter 5.3

Significance testing

Overview

When we gather data through a study, we need to assess whether the observed relationship (e.g. between variables) or a difference (e.g. between means) in a sample occurred by pure chance. Statistical significance testing is the tool used to determine whether the outcome of a study is the result of a relationship between specific factors or due to chance.

Every test of significance begins with a hypothesis. A statistical hypothesis is an assumption about a population parameter. This assumption may or may not be true.

There are two types of statistical hypotheses.

- *Null hypothesis:* the null hypothesis, denoted by H_0, is a statistical hypothesis that is tested for possible rejection under the assumption that it is true. The null hypothesis would be stated as 'There is no mean difference between groups' or 'There is no correlation between variables'.
- *Alternative hypothesis:* the alternative hypothesis, denoted by H_1 or H_a, is the hypothesis that sample observations are influenced by some non-random cause. This would be stated as 'There is a (significant) mean difference between groups', or 'There is a (significant) correlation between variables'.

It is important to understand that the *null hypothesis can never be proven*. A set of data can only reject a null hypothesis or fail to reject it.

Significance testing process

A formal process must be followed in order to determine whether or not to reject the null hypothesis.

This process seeks to answer these questions:

- What are the null hypothesis and the alternative hypothesis?
- Which test statistic is appropriate, and what is the probability distribution?
- What is the required level of significance?
- What is the decision rule?
- Do we reject or fail to reject the null hypothesis?

What are the null hypothesis and the alternative hypothesis?

The null hypothesis is the statement that will be tested. In hypothesis testing, the null hypothesis is initially regarded to be true, until we gather enough proof to either reject the null hypothesis, or fail to reject the null hypothesis. The alternative hypothesis is a statement that will be accepted as a result of the null hypothesis being rejected.

Which test statistic is appropriate, and what is the probability distribution?

We must choose an appropriate test statistic. In hypothesis testing, a test statistic is defined as a quantity taken from a sample that is used as the basis for testing the null hypothesis (rejecting or failing to reject the null).

Calculating a test statistic will vary based on our choice of probability distribution (for example, *t*-test, *z*-value).

What is the required level of significance?

First, we must consider the 2 types of errors which can occur. A type I error is defined as rejecting the null hypothesis when it is true. A type II error is defined as not rejecting the null hypothesis when it is false.

The significance level is the probability of making a type I error, or the probability that we will reject the null hypothesis when it is true. So if we choose a significance level of 0.05, it means there is a 5% chance of making a type I error. A 0.01 significance level means there is just a 1% chance of making a type I error.

One important concept in significance testing is whether you use a one-tailed or two-tailed test of significance. The answer is that it depends on your hypothesis. When your research hypothesis states the direction of the difference or relationship, then you use a one-tailed probability. For example, a one-tailed test would be used to test these null hypotheses: Superman is not stronger than the average person. In this case, the null hypothesis (indirectly) predicts the direction of the difference. A two-tailed test would be used if the null hypotheses stated: There is no difference in strength between Superman and the average person. The one-tailed probability is exactly half the value of the two-tailed probability.

Do we reject or fail to reject the null hypothesis?

Based on the sample data, what is the value of the test statistic? If the probability value ≤ significance level then we reject the null hypothesis and conclude that the research finding is statistically significant.

If the probability value > significance level then we fail to reject the null hypothesis and conclude that the research finding is not statistically significant (see Box 5.4.1).

Box 5.4.1 Interpreting results

If: probability value ≤0.05.
Then: reject the null hypothesis.
And: conclude that the finding is statistically significant.

If: probability value >0.05.
Then: fail to reject the null hypothesis.
And: conclude that the research finding is not statistically significant.

Type I and Type II error

Overview

We must accept some level of error in every study. Indeed, for all studies we predetermine what is the acceptable level of error, typically setting significance thresholds of 0.05 or 0.01. There are two kinds of errors that can be made in significance testing:

- A true null hypothesis can be incorrectly rejected
- A false null hypothesis can fail to be rejected.

The former error is called a Type I error, and the latter error is called a Type II error.

Understanding Type I Type II error

A Type I error, also known as a false positive, occurs when the results of research show that a difference exists, but in reality there is no difference.

A Type II error, also known as a false negative, occurs when the results of research show that no difference exists but in reality there is a difference. These two types of errors are shown in Fig. 5.4.1.

	Null Hypothesis True	Null Hypothesis False
Reject Null Hypothesis	Type I Error	Correct
Accept Null Hypothesis	Correct	Type II Error

Fig. 5.4.1 Type I and Type II errors.

The significance level of a test equals the probability of occurrence of a result as extreme or more extreme than that observed, if the null hypothesis were true. Therefore the probability that we commit a Type I error, denoted by the Greek letter alpha (α), is equal to the significance level of the test (see Box 5.4.1).

Box 5.4.1 Example

In a study we set α at 0.05. We are therefore saying that we will accept 5% error. This means that if the study were to be conducted 100 times, we would expect to identify the correct outcome in 95 studies, and the incorrect one in 5 studies. However, as we generally only carry out any given study once, we do not know if any result we get falls into the 5% error category.

The rate of the type II error is denoted by the Greek letter beta (β) and is related to the power of a test (which equals 1-β).

Relationship with power

There is a relationship between these two measures. As you increase power you increase the chances that you are going to find an effect if it's there. However, if you increase the chances of this, you must at the same time be increasing the chances of making a Type I error!

It is therefore clear that if we wish to reduce the Type I error rate, we can reduce the level of acceptable error (e.g. reduce α from 0.05 to 0.01). Lowering α has the direct effect of lowering the power of the study, thereby increasing the chance of a Type II error. In other words, the greater the chances of a Type I error, the less likely a Type II error, and vice versa. Since we usually want high power *and* low Type I error, one should be able to appreciate that there is built-in tension here.

Chapter 5.5

Confidence intervals

Overview

A confidence interval is a range of plausible values that accounts for uncertainty in a statistical estimate. In simple terms a confidence interval (CI) calculated for a measure of treatment effect shows the range within which the true treatment effect is likely to lie (see Box 5.5.1).

> ### Box 5.5.1 Example
> In a study comparing 2 diabetes therapies, a mean difference in reduction in HbA1c of 0.8% was demonstrated. The 95% CI is 0.6%–1.0%.

Therefore, while the mean difference is 0.8%, this is unlikely to be the true value. However, we can be 95% confident that the true value lies between 0.6% and 1.0%.

Therefore, it is clear that a narrower CI suggests higher precision as we can specify plausible values to within a narrow range. Conversely, a wider interval implies poorer precision, as we can only specify plausible values to a broader range, which may be less informative.

How to interpret a confidence interval

There are 2 important things to consider when interpreting a CI:
- Does the CI include the point of no effect:
  - 0 if looking for differences.
  - 1 if looking at a ratio.
- Does the interval lie within the area of no clinical significance?

In the example above, we are looking at differences, so the point of no effect is zero. Fig. 5.5.1 shows this graphically.

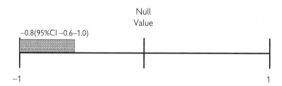

Fig. 5.5.1 CI showing statistical significance.

As this value does not contain the point of no effect, this suggests that this is a statistically significant effect.

Now we should consider whether this lies within the area of clinical insignificance. Clinical insignificance represents values that you would not lead you to change your current practice. Choosing this is not a statistical decision, but rather one based on knowledge of the range of possible treatments, their costs, and their side effects. In the case above we could decide that any improvement less than 0.4% would not be clinically significant, even if it were statistically significant.

We could therefore show this graphically in Fig. 5.5.2.

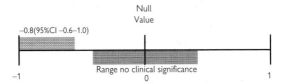

Fig. 5.5.2 CI showing no statistical or clinical significance.

The result therefore lies outside the range of no clinical significance. This suggests that the result is not only statistically significant, but also clinically significant.

If the result had been different, for instance −0.3 (95% CI −0.1, −0.5) then the situation would be as demonstrated in Fig. 5.5.3.

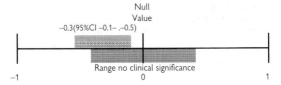

Fig. 5.5.3 CI showing statistical significance but not clinical significance.

This suggests that while the result remains statistically significant, it may or may not be clinically significant. In this case the study may have been underpowered as the width of your CI goes down as the sample size goes up.

Calculating confidence intervals

In order to generate a CI, we need to define the appropriate range. We use what are called critical values. These are usually taken from the standard normal distribution whether the confidence interval is for a mean, proportion, or a rate. On this scale, 95% of the probability is contained between z values of −1.96 and +1.96 (see Fig. 5.5.4). These are the critical values most widely used for calculating confidence limits.

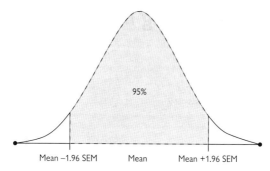

Fig. 5.5.4 CI in normal distribution.

In a sample mean follows a normal distribution, 95% of the distribution of sample means will lie within 1.96 standard deviations (SD) of the population mean. If we only have a single sample, we call this the sample error of the mean (SEM).

Therefore, the 95%CI is usually calculated as ($\overline{X}$ −1.96 SEM, $\overline{X}$ +1.96 SEM).

If we compute a proportion, p, from a sample, the standard error of that proportion would be:

$$\sqrt{\frac{p \times (1-p)}{n}}$$

If we are using odds ratios, the letters a, b, c, and d represent the frequency counts in a 2×2 table:

a b

c d

then the odds ratio would be ad/bc. The odds ratio is skewed, so we cannot easily compute a standard error for the odds ratio itself. We can, however, find a standard error for the natural logarithm of the odds ratio. It is simply:

$$\sqrt{\frac{1}{a} + \frac{1}{b} + \frac{1}{c} + \frac{1}{d}}$$

If data are not normally distributed and/or we do not know the sample variance, the sample mean follows a t distribution. Therefore, the 95% CI is:

($\overline{X}$ −($t_{0.05}$ SEM), $\overline{X}$ +($t_{0.05}$ SEM)) where $t_{0.05}$ is the percentile of the t-distribution with n−1 degrees of freedom.

Chapter 5.6

Minimizing bias

Overview

The term 'bias' describes the systematic tendency of any factors associated with the design, conduct, analysis, and interpretation of the results of clinical trials to make the estimate of a treatment effect deviate from its true value. It is important to identify potential sources of bias as completely as possible so that attempts to limit such bias may be made. The presence of bias may seriously compromise the ability to draw valid conclusions from clinical trials.

Bias arises from:
- *The design of the trial:* for example, an assignment of treatments such that subjects at lower risk are systematically assigned to one treatment.
- *The conduct and analysis of a clinical trial:* for example, protocol violations and exclusion of subjects from analysis based upon knowledge of subject outcomes.

Types of bias

There are many different types of biases described in the research literature. The most common categories of bias that can affect the validity of research include:
- *Selection biases:* may result in the subjects in the sample being unrepresentative of the population of interest.
- *Measurement biases:* includes issues related to how the outcome of interest was measured.
- *Intervention (exposure) biases:* involves differences in how the treatment or intervention was carried out, or how subjects were exposed to the factor of interest.

Minimizing bias

The most important design techniques for avoiding bias in clinical trials are blinding and randomization, and these should be normal features of most controlled clinical trials intended to be included in a marketing application.

Blinding

The essential aim of blinding is to prevent identification of the treatments until all opportunities for bias have passed. This will limit the occurrence of conscious and unconscious bias in the conduct and interpretation of a clinical trial arising from:
- The influence which the knowledge of treatment may have on the recruitment and allocation of subjects, their subsequent care.
- The attitudes of subjects to the treatments.
- The assessment of end-points.
- The handling of withdrawals.
- The exclusion of data from analysis.

A double-blind trial is one in which neither the subject nor any of the investigator or sponsor staff who are involved in the treatment or clinical evaluation of the subjects are aware of the treatment received.

This level of blinding is maintained throughout the conduct of the trial. Difficulties in achieving the double-blind ideal can arise:
• The treatments may be of a completely different nature, for example, surgery and drug therapy.
• Two drugs may have different formulations.
• The daily pattern of administration of two treatments may differ.

Extensive efforts should be made to overcome these difficulties.

Breaking the blind (for a single subject) should be considered only when knowledge of the treatment assignment is deemed essential by the subject's physician for the subject's care.

Randomization

Randomization introduces a deliberate element of chance into the assignment of treatments to subjects in a clinical trial. It provides a sound statistical basis for the quantitative evaluation of the evidence relating to treatment effects.

In combination with blinding, randomization helps to avoid possible bias in the selection and allocation of subjects arising from the predictability of treatment assignments.

The common types of randomization include:
• *Simple randomization:* this method is equivalent to tossing a coin for each subject that enters a trial. The random number generator is generally used. However, it can get imbalanced in treatment assignment, especially in smaller trials.
• *Block randomization:* some advantages can generally be gained by randomizing subjects in blocks. This helps to increase the comparability of the treatment groups, particularly when subject characteristics may change over time, as a result, for example, of changes in recruitment policy. It also provides a better guarantee that the treatment groups will be of nearly equal size.
• *Stratified randomization:* stratified randomization is used to ensure that equal numbers of participants with a characteristic thought to affect prognosis or response to the intervention will be allocated to each comparison group.
• *Unequal randomization:* most randomized trials allocate equal numbers of patients to experimental and control groups. However, this may not be ethically/practically feasible, and you may wish to randomize in an alternative ratio, e.g. 2:1 to limit the number of people in a placebo arm.

Further reading

ICH Topic E9 (1998). Statistical principles for clinical trials. CPMP/ICH/363/96. Available at: 🔊 http://www.emea.europa.eu/docs/en_GB/document_library/Scientific_guideline/2009/09/WC500002928.pdf

Paired and unpaired *t*-tests

Overview

A *t*-test is a very standard statistical test to compare the means of two groups. As other kinds of statistical test do, a *t*-test makes some assumptions. The first important assumption is that the distribution of the population of your sample data is normal. The *t*-distribution is symmetric and bell-shaped, like the normal distribution, but has heavier tails, meaning that it is more prone to producing values that fall far from its mean.

There is one important distinction you need to understand in a *t*-test: the difference between paired and unpaired tests.

Paired test

In a paired test, or 'repeated samples *t*-test,' the data is collected from subjects measured at two different points wherein each subject has two measurements which are done before and after the treatment. This is also known as the repeated samples *t*-test.

An example would be comparing the weight loss of a group of people who are being put on a strict diet. These people are weighed before they are started with the new diet and are again tested after they have been on the new diet for a period of time. The results of both tests given to the same set group of people determine how much weight they have lost while on the special diet.

Unpaired test

The unpaired, or 'independent samples' *t*-test is used when two separate sets of independent and identically distributed samples are obtained, one from each of the two populations being compared. For example, suppose we are evaluating the effect of cholesterol lowering treatment, and we enroll 100 subjects into our study, and then randomize 50 subjects to the treatment group and 50 subjects to the control group. In this case, we have two independent samples and would use the unpaired form of the *t*-test. Therefore, we would calculate the sample means within the treated and untreated groups of subjects, and compare these means with each other.

A paired test, therefore, is a test of the null hypothesis that the means of two groups of subjects that are normally distributed are equal; while an unpaired test is the test of the null hypothesis that two responses which are measured in the same unit have a difference with a mean value of zero.

Both tests assume that all data that have been analysed are normally distributed. Paired *t*-tests are more comprehensive and compelling than unpaired *t*-tests because they are carried out with subjects that have similar characteristics.

Summary

- A paired test is the test of the null hypothesis that the means of two subjects are equal, while an unpaired test is the test of the null hypothesis that the difference between subjects has the mean value of zero.
- A paired test is also known as a repeated samples *t*-test, while an unpaired test is also known as a student's *t*-test.
- A paired test is carried out on subjects that are similar or paired before data is collected and two tests are carried out before and after a treatment, while an unpaired test is done on two independent subjects.

Parametric and non-parametric tests

Overview

In clinical research, continuous data is the type that arises most frequently. Examples include blood pressure, ejection fraction, and serum cholesterol. Methods for analysing continuous data fall into two classes, distinguished by whether or not they make assumptions about the distribution of the data. Methods that use distributional assumptions are called parametric methods. Parametric data has an underlying normal distribution, which allows for more conclusions to be drawn as the shape can be mathematically described. Anything else is non-parametric—see Table 5.8.1 for a summary.

Table 5.8.1 Summary of parametric and non-parametric test features

	Parametric	Non-parametric
Assumed distribution	Normal	Any
Assumed variance	Homogeneous	Any
Typical data	Ratio or Interval	Ordinal or Nominal
Data set relationships	Independent	Any
Usual central measure	Mean	Median
Benefits	Can draw more conclusions	Simplicity; less affected by outliers

Parametric methods

Frequently used parametric methods include:
- *t*-tests.
- Analysis of variance for comparing groups.
- Least squares regression and correlation for studying the relation between variables.

All of the common parametric methods assume that in some way the data follow a normal distribution and also that the spread of the data (variance) is uniform either between groups or across the range being studied. For example, the two sample *t*-test assumes that the two samples of observations come from populations that have normal distributions with the same standard deviation. The importance of the assumptions for *t* methods diminishes as sample size increases.

Alternative methods, such as the sign test, Mann–Whitney test, and rank correlation, do not require the data to follow a particular distribution. They work by using the rank order of observations, rather than the measurements themselves.

Non-parametric methods

Methods that do not require us to make distributional assumptions about the data, such as the rank methods, are called non-parametric methods.

Non-parametric methods are most often used to analyse data, which are not normally distributed. Skewed data are frequently analysed by non-parametric methods, although data transformation can often make the data suitable for parametric analyses.

Examples of non-parametric tests are:
• Wilcoxon signed rank test.
• Whitney–Mann–Wilcoxon (WMW) test.
• Kruskal–Wallis (KW) test.
• Friedman's test.

Data that are scores, rather than measurements may have many possible values, such as quality of life scales or data from visual analogue scales, while others have only a few possible values, such as Apgar scores or stage of disease. Scores with many values are often analysed using parametric methods, whereas those with few values tend to be analysed using rank methods.

To compensate for the advantage of being free of assumptions about the distribution of the data, rank methods have the disadvantage that they are mainly suited to hypothesis testing and no useful estimate is obtained, such as the average difference between two groups.

The choice of approach may also be related to sample size, as the distributional assumptions are more important for small samples.

Patient reported outcomes

Overview

- A patient reported outcome (PRO) is any report of the status of a patient's health condition that comes directly from the patient, without interpretation of the patient's response by a clinician or anyone else.
- In clinical trials, a PRO instrument is advised when measuring a concept best known by the patient or best measured from the patient perspective. These include a patient's symptoms, signs, or an aspect of functioning directly related to disease status.
- Generally, findings measured by a well-defined and reliable PRO instrument in appropriately designed investigations can be used to support a claim in medical product labelling if the claim is consistent with the instrument's documented measurement capability.

Choice of patient reported outcome instrument

Researchers planning to use a PRO instrument in support of a product claim should determine whether an adequate PRO instrument exists to assess the measure of interest. If it does not, a new PRO instrument can be developed. In some situations, the new instrument can be developed by modifying an existing instrument.

The adequacy of any PRO instrument to support medical product labelling claims depends whether the following are satisfactory.

Reliability

- *Test-retest or intra-interviewer reliability:* stability of scores over time when no change is expected in the concept of interest.
- *Internal consistency:* extent to which items comprising a scale measure the same concept.
- *Inter-interviewer reliability:* extent to which items comprising a scale measure the same concept.

Validity

- *Content validity:* evidence that the instrument measures the concept of interest including evidence from qualitative studies that the items and domains of an instrument are appropriate and comprehensive relative to its intended measurement concept, population, and use.
- *Construct validity:* evidence that relationships among items, domains, and concepts conform to *a priori* hypotheses concerning logical relationships that should exist with measures of related concepts or scores produced in similar or diverse patient groups.

Ability to detect change

Evidence that a PRO instrument can identify differences in scores over time in individuals or groups who have changed with respect to the measurement concept.

Clinical trial design with patient reported outcomes

General protocol considerations

If the PRO measurement goal is to support licensing, this should be stated as a specific clinical trial objective or hypothesis. Open-label clinical trials are rarely adequate to support this. There should be standardization in how PRO and other clinical assessments are administered. Missing data is a major challenge and, therefore, the protocol should describe how missing data will be handled in the analysis.

Frequency of assessments

Some diseases, conditions, or clinical trial designs may necessitate more than one baseline assessment and several PRO assessments during treatment.

Clinical trial duration

It is important to consider whether the clinical trial's duration is of adequate length to support the proposed claim and assess a durable outcome in the disease or condition being studied. Generally, duration of follow-up with a PRO assessment should be the same as for other measures of effectiveness.

Further reading

FDA (2009). Guidance for Industry. Patient-reported outcome measures: use in medical product development to support labelling claims.

Chapter 5.10

Health-related quality of life

Overview

In the context of drug approval, health-related quality of life (HRQL) is considered to represent a specific type/subset of PROs, distinguished by its multi-dimensionality. Indeed, HRQL is a broad concept which can be defined as the patient's subjective perception of the impact of his disease and its treatment(s) on his daily life, physical, psychological, and social functioning and well-being.

The definition of HRQL has as a common basis the definition of health given by the WHO in 1948 as a state of total physical, mental, and social well-being and not simply the absence of disease.

The basis for the approval of a new medicinal product is its efficacy and safety. Therefore, in the drug evaluation process, the first step is to assess efficacy and safety. However, there is an increasing need to measure the effect of the medicinal product on HRQL. A claim about improvement in HRQL needs to be supported by data collected by instruments validated for use in the corresponding condition. In order to approve a global claim that a product 'improves HRQL,' it would be necessary to demonstrate robust improvements in all or most of these domains.

The claim in the SmPC with the respect to HRQL will be considered depending on the strength of the evidence and the relevance of the finding. The strength of the evidence should be based on the:
- Rationale for HRQL assessment in the context of the disease or medicinal product.
- Justification of the choice of the HRQL questionnaire(s).
- Objectives of HRQL assessment.
- Hypotheses of HRQL changes.
- Evidence of validation (and of cultural adaptation/translation if applicable) of the HRQL questionnaire.
- Adequacy of the statistical analysis plan.
- Relevance of observed changes.

Study design for health-related quality of life assessment

The validation of HRQL instrument should ideally have been completed before its use in therapeutic confirmatory trials.

If the HRQL instrument planned to be used is not validated (or is insufficiently validated), it is recommended to test it first in the therapeutic exploratory trials setting before use in therapeutic confirmatory trials. If HRQL is planned to be assessed, it should be implemented in the drug development plan as early as possible.

Regarding the timing of HRQL assessment related to the marketing authorization, broadly two situations may be met:
- The medicinal product has no MA. A company may choose to study HRQL simultaneously with efficacy/safety. In this case, the efficacy endpoint and HRQL may be co-primary endpoints or HRQL may be a secondary endpoint.

- Test drug has obtained MA or HRQL is decided to be studied once efficacy and safety of the test drug have already been shown in the target population. In this situation, it may be difficult to perform a study vs. placebo if the product has already shown efficacy and obtained MA. HRQL change due to the test drug may be compared with HRQL change due to an active comparator.

In severe, life-threatening diseases, HRQL may provide important information. There must be confidence that the observed HRQL benefit is achieved without any reduction in efficacy. The impossibility of blinding in some studies may create bias. Therefore, open-label studies are not recommended.

In chronic non-life-threatening conditions requiring long-term treatments, the information on HRQL might be important for the choice of one medicinal product over the other in the current clinical practice.

Further reading

Committee for Medicinal Products for Human Use (CHMP). Reflection paper on the regulatory guidance for the use of health related quality of life measures in the evaluation of medicinal products. EMEA/CHMP/EWP/139391/2004. Available at: ℞ http://www.ispor.org/workpaper/emea-hrql-guidance.pdf

Clinical interpretation of trial results

Outcomes of randomized trials

Parallel group randomized controlled trials (RCTs) are diverse in their design and international guidelines for the reporting of such studies have recently been updated (CONSORT). The CONSORT statement is an evidence-based 25-item checklist (see Table 5.11.1) and flow diagram, representing the minimum set of requirements for reporting RCTs. Clinical trial outcome variables may take various forms, each having their appropriate methods of statistical analysis:

- Counts, e.g. deaths.
- Continuous variables, e.g. blood pressure.
- Failure time data, e.g. survival, disease-free survival.

After conventional statistical analysis, results will be expressed as:

- A point estimate of treatment effect, e.g. odds ratio of death, difference in mean blood pressure, difference in mean survival time.
- The range of uncertainty about that estimate, e.g. the 95% CI.
- A significance test, the probability of observing such a result on the assumption (the null hypothesis) that there is no true treatment effect, the p-value.

For all clinical trials, there are the same criteria to be used when judging whether their results should be applied in clinical practice.

Table 5.11.1 CONSORT checklist items

Item	Checklist item
1a	Identification as a randomized trial in the title
1b	Structured summary of trial design, methods, results, and conclusions
2a	Background and objectives—scientific background and explanation of rationale
2b	Specific objectives or hypotheses
3a	Trial design—description of trial design (such as parallel, factorial) including allocation ratio
3b	Important changes to methods after trial commencement (such as eligibility criteria), with reasons
4a	Participants—eligibility criteria for participants
4b	Settings and locations where the data were collected
5	Interventions—the interventions for each group with sufficient details to allow replication, including how and when they were actually administered
6a	Outcomes—completely defined pre-specified primary and secondary outcome measures, including how and when they were assessed
6b	Any changes to trial outcomes after the trial commenced, with reasons
7a	Sample size—how sample size was determined

(Continued)

Table 5.11.1 (*Continued*)

Item	Checklist item
7b	When applicable, explanation of any interim analyses and stopping guidelines
8a	Randomization—sequence generation; method used to generate the random allocation sequence
8b	Type of randomization; details of any restriction (such as blocking and block size)
9	Allocation concealment mechanism—mechanism used to implement the random allocation sequence (such as sequentially numbered containers), describing any steps taken to conceal the sequence until interventions were assigned
10	Implementation—who generated the random allocation sequence, who enrolled participants, and who assigned participants to interventions
11a	Blinding—if done, who was blinded after assignment to interventions (for example, participants, care providers, those assessing outcomes) and how
11b	If relevant, description of the similarity of interventions
12a	Statistical methods—statistical methods used to compare groups for primary and secondary outcomes
12b	Methods for additional analyses, such as subgroup analyses and adjusted analyses
13a	Participant flow (a diagram is strongly recommended)—for each group, the numbers of participants who were randomly assigned, received intended treatment, and were analysed for the primary outcome
13b	For each group, losses and exclusions after randomization, together with reasons
14a	Recruitment—dates defining the periods of recruitment and follow-up
14b	Why the trial ended or was stopped
15	Baseline data—a table showing baseline demographic and clinical characteristics for each group
16	Numbers analysed—for each group, number of participants (denominator) included in each analysis and whether the analysis was by original assigned groups
17a	Outcomes and estimation—for each primary and secondary outcome, results for each group, and the estimated effect size and its precision (such as 95% confidence interval)
17b	For binary outcomes, presentation of both absolute and relative effect sizes is recommended
18	Ancillary analyses—results of any other analyses performed, including subgroup analyses and adjusted analyses, distinguishing pre-specified from exploratory

(*Continued*)

Table 5.11.1 (Continued)

Item	Checklist item
19	Harms—all important harms or unintended effects in each group
20	Limitations—trial limitations, addressing sources of potential bias, imprecision, and, if relevant, multiplicity of analyses
21	Generalizability—generalizability (external validity, applicability) of the trial findings
22	Interpretation—interpretation consistent with results, balancing benefits and harms, and considering other relevant evidence
23	Registration—registration number and name of trial registry
24	Protocol—where the full trial protocol can be accessed, if available
25	Funding—sources of funding and other support (such as supply of drugs), role of funders

Reproduced under a Creative Commons licence from Schultz KF, Altman DG, Moher D, for the CONSORT Group. CONSORT 2010 Statement: updated guidelines for reporting parallel group randomized trials. BMJ 2010; 340:c332. Available at: ℘ http://www.consort-statement.org/

Internal validity (lack of bias)

Randomization should ensure that characteristics likely to influence outcome, such as age or disease severity, are distributed similarly in the comparison groups. Observed outcome differences should then be unbiased: due either to a true treatment effect or to the 'play of chance' (indicated by the result of the significance test or the confidence interval). Bias can arise in many ways:

• Poorly concealed randomization, allowing conscious or unconscious selection of subjects (this can be looked for by comparing the baseline characteristics of the randomized groups).
• Differential losses to follow up, or exclusion from analysis, in treatment-related ways, e.g. side effects, inefficacy, poor compliance.
• Differences in follow up, such as frequency of review, or differing quality of care.
• Biased assessment of outcome measures when treatment allocation is known or can be guessed.
• Data-derived analyses, i.e. analyses not specified in advance as primary outcomes of interest, but suggested by the observed findings. Sub-group analyses, unless pre-specified in the design, should be considered as exploratory rather than hypothesis-testing.

External validity (generalizability)

To what clinical population of patients does this trial sample relate? Two information sources can shed light on this:

- The inclusion and exclusion criteria specified in the protocol.
- The reported characteristics of the patients actually randomized, in particular age and gender distribution, disease severity and duration, and concurrent illness and treatment.

Is it appropriate to generalize the findings to patients of a different age or health status to those included in the trial? This is usually a matter of clinical judgement; patients recruited in trials are often younger and fitter than average.

Benefit and harm

- Are the outcomes clinically relevant (e.g. survival, morbidity) or surrogates (e.g. change in biochemical parameters)?
- Have adverse outcomes been recorded and presented fully?
- Are the effects reported of a magnitude to be clinically significant as well as statistically significant?
- How many patients would need to be treated to benefit one patient (NNT; number needed to treat)?

Plausibility and consistency

- Are the findings consistent with the known mechanism of action of the treatment?
- Are they consistent with findings of other trials of the same intervention?
- Have the findings been included in a systematic review of evidence, including meta-analysis where feasible?

The weight of the evidence

No trial is perfect. Where possible sources of bias are identified, one must ask the direction in which they might have skewed the results and the likely scale of their impact. The less the supportive evidence of mechanism and external corroboration, the more care is needed to look for an effect of bias on an apparently positive trial outcome. Small trials are statistically more likely than large ones to miss a true treatment effect (Type II error) or to generate an extreme chance positive result highlighted by publication bias. When methodological and statistical aspects have been scrutinized, clinical judgement must be applied to the applicability of the results to routine care.

Further reading

Schultz KF, Altman DG, Moher D, for the CONSORT Group. CONSORT 2010 Statement: updated guidelines for reporting parallel group randomised trials. *BMJ* 2010; **340**: c332. Available at: ℘ http://www.consort-statement.org/

Clinical study report

Overview

The ICH Harmonised Tripartite Guideline E3 provides guidance on the structure and content of clinical study reports to allow the compilation of a single core clinical study report acceptable to all regulatory authorities of the ICH regions. The aim is to reduce post-submission requests for data clarification and analyses as much as possible.

The clinical study report should also ensure that there is no ambiguity in how the study was conducted. Therefore, it should provide:

• The design features of the study, why they were chosen.
• Information on the plan, methods and conduct of the study.
• Individual patient data, including the demographic and baseline data.
• Details of analytical methods, to allow replication of the analyses, should the authorities wish to do so.

Structure of the full integrated report

The structure of the full integrated report is shown in Box 5.12.1.

Each report should consider all of the topics described, although the specific sequence and grouping of topics may be changed if alternatives are more logical for a particular study. The protocol may be restated in order to fulfil the requirement of the detailed description of how the study was carried out. However, it is important to clarify features of the study that are not well-described in the protocol and any deviations from the protocol.

The report should include the detailed discussion of individual adverse events or laboratory abnormalities. The report should describe, where possible, potentially predictive characteristics of the study population.

Data should be presented in the report at appropriate levels of detail. Therefore, overall summary figures and tables for important demographic, efficacy and safety variables may be placed in the text to illustrate key points, with other summary figures, tables, and listings for demographic, efficacy, and safety variables being provided in section 14.

Alternative structure

In the case of very large trials, this structure may not be practical. When reporting such trials an appropriate format should be agreed with the regulators.

However, in some cases an abbreviated report may be acceptable using summarized data or with some sections deleted. This may be the case for:

• Uncontrolled studies.
• Studies not designed to establish efficacy.
• Flawed or aborted studies.
• Controlled studies that examine conditions clearly unrelated to those for which a claim is made.

Box 5.12.1 Structure of clinical study report
1. Title.
2. Synopsis.
3. Table of contents for the individual clinical study report.
4. List of abbreviations and definition of terms.
5. Ethics.
6. Investigators and study administrative structure.
7. Introduction.
8. Study objectives.
9. Investigational plan.
10. Study patients.
11. Efficacy evaluation.
12. Safety evaluation.
13. Discussion and overall conclusions.
14. Tables, figures and graphs referred to but not included in the text.
15. Reference list.
16. Appendices.

However, a full description of safety aspects should be included in these cases. If an abbreviated report is submitted, there should be enough detail of design and results to allow the regulatory authority to determine whether a full report is needed.

Further reading

International Conference on Harmonisation of Technical Requirements for Registration of Pharmaceuticals for Human Use: ICH Harmonised Tripartite Guideline 'Structure and Content of Clinical Study Reports'. E3 Current *Step 4* version dated 30 November 1995.

Chapter 5.13

Issues with making trial results available

Overview

The ethical interpretation and publication of research results are essential to ensure the validity, timeliness, and accessibility of new knowledge for patients, physicians, and regulatory agencies. Failure to adhere to ethical principles may cause adverse outcomes for patients because of overestimation of benefit, underestimation of harm, and lack of timely awareness of benefit or harm.

Publication bias

The persistent gap between the number of trials conducted and the number for which results are publicly available has been well-documented.

This publication bias is a result of statistically significant, 'positive' results being:
- More likely to be published (publication bias).
- More likely to be published rapidly (time lag bias).
- More likely to be published in English (language bias).
- More likely to be published more than once (multiple publication bias).
- More likely to be cited by others (citation bias).

All of these reporting biases make positive studies easier to find than those with non-significant and negative results. Failing to publish negative findings could thus contribute to a series of risks, including:
- Misinformed clinical decision making based on incomplete or skewed data.
- Inappropriate and potentially harmful clinical practices and injury to health.
- Needless and wasteful duplication of research with associated risks to participants.
- Fraud or deception in the clinical trials process.
- Erosion of public trust and accountability in research.

If research findings are not disseminated their value may be diminished or lost, betraying the contributions and sacrifices of participants. For this reason, researchers and institutions have an ethical responsibility to make reasonable efforts to publicly disseminate the findings of clinical trials.

Trial registries

There is therefore a need for transparency in clinical research. This transparency extends from the documentation of the existence of a trial to the full disclosure of the results. Trial registries make public a summary of protocol details at trial initiation (see Fig. 5.13.1). The NIH has maintained ClinicalTrials.gov, the largest single registry of clinical trials, since 2000. The International Committee of Medical Journal Editors (ICMJE) also requires prospective trial registration as a pre-condition for publication, effective September 2005.

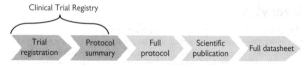

Fig. 5.13.1 Details in CT registry.

However, clinical trial registries do not currently require dissemination of findings.

On 27 September 2007, the FDA Amendments Act was enacted, which defines the scope of required registrations at ClinicalTrials.gov and also calls on the NIH to augment ClinicalTrials.gov to include a 'basic results' database (see Box 5.13.1).

Box 5.13.1 Data elements in a 'basic results' database

- Participant demographics.
- Baseline characteristics.
- Primary and secondary outcomes.
- Statistical analyses.
- Disclosure of agreements between sponsors and non-employees restricting researchers from disseminating results at scientific forums.

Summary

When researchers embark on a clinical trial, they make a commitment to conduct the trial and to report the findings in accordance with basic ethical principles. This includes preserving the accuracy of the results and making both positive and negative results available. However, much research remains unpublished. Selective reporting, regardless of the reason for it, leads to an incomplete and potentially biased view of a trial and its results.

Further reading

Easterbrook PJ, Berlin JA, Gopalan R, Matthews DR (1991). Publication bias in clinical research. *The Lancet.* **337**: 867.

Cochrane Collaboration open learning materials. Available at: ℘ http://www.cochrane-net.org/openlearning/html/mod15-2.htm

DeAngelis CD, Drazen JM, Frizelle FA, *et al.* (2004). Clinical trial registration: a statement from the International Committee of Medical Journal Editors. *J Am Med Ass* **292**: 1363.

Interim analysis

Overview

Considerations for interim analysis are multiple, as are the range of studies where interim analyses are performed. Whilst it is a useful tool when analysing exploratory studies and taking decisions such as adding or removing dose levels, examining safety parameters, etc., when it comes to large phase III efficacy and safety programmes, it can be fraught with danger, leaving underpowered results where no meaningful conclusions can be drawn with respect to efficacy or safety (see Table 5.14.1).

Limitations and advantages of interim analysis

See Table 5.14.1.

Table 5.14.1 Limitations and advantages of interim analysis

Consequences of interim analysis	Uses	Limitations
Protocol modification	Might help to answer the primary study question and to generate new hypotheses	Requires extra methodological and statistical safeguards
Early termination for efficacy	Might speed up dissemination of effective treatments. Might fulfil an ethical obligation to protect trial participants	Estimate of treatment effect is imprecise and will, on average, be falsely inflated. Information on secondary outcomes diminishes. Benefit–risk ratio might be difficult to assess
Early termination for harm	Protection of trial participants. Avoidance of further patient exposure to harmful treatments	Risks abandonment of a treatment that might be beneficial. Information on primary and secondary outcomes diminishes
Early termination for futility	Saves resources that could be used on more promising research	Leaves primary study question unanswered. Information on secondary outcomes diminishes. Estimate of treatment effect is imprecise and might be biased downward. Interpretation of trial might become more complex

(Continued)

Table 5.14.1 (Continued)

Consequences of interim analysis	Uses	Limitations
Publication of interim results whilst trial is ongoing	Open disclosure of total available evidence. Might protect the trial's integrity	Might create uncertainty. Might lead to a loss of power of the on-going study Might compromise the trial's integrity

Summary points

- Prospectively plan interim analyses wherever possible.
- If you decide to plan an interim analysis *ad hoc*, make sure that it is the best decision.
- Take both the uses and limitations into account when considering the reasons for interim analysis.
- Bear in mind that it may render the results of your study interpretable with respect to clinical practice.

Further reading

℘ http://clinicalevidence.bmj.com/downloads/15-08-07.pdf

Chapter 5.15

Data management

Overview

As with many other aspects of clinical trials, the collection and management of data must be carefully planned before the trial begins. It is not sufficient to collect data and decide at a later stage, possibly after the trial has finished, how the database is to be managed. The processes for handling the clinical trial data should be discussed in advance by the full clinical trial team where each of the important functions are represented (e.g. clinical, statistical, statistical programming, data management, coding, and monitoring) to ensure that the final database is adequate for the statistical analyses required to address the objectives of the study. Data collection should be limited to information which is necessary for the analysis, inference, and reporting of the study. In this way data management resources can be focused on providing relevant data of high quality.

During planning, the following aspects require careful consideration:
- The number of variables to be collected and the frequency of data collection.
- How to promote the accuracy of recording key variables.
- How to promote the completeness of important data.
- How to verify the internal consistency of the patient data recorded within the database.

The focus of the data checking procedures should be on the key information to be collected. Previous experience gained from similar trials will provide useful information about what can be expected in terms of the quality of the data and the quantity likely to be missing or incorrect.

It is highly unlikely that all data requested on the case report form will be accurately and fully completed at the initial entry of the data whether paper or electronic collection is used. Having accepted that the database is almost certain to have some missing information, the algorithms to be programmed to handle this must be clearly described in the statistical analysis plan which should be finalized before the database is locked and the study unblinded.

Coding of data

The collection of certain information may be simplified by offering a series of alternatives either on the paper case report form or in a pull-down menu when electronic data capture is being used. In order to simplify the terminology and therefore ensure that data may be summarized it is common practice to use a recognized coding system or dictionary for medications (e.g. WHO Drug) and for medical conditions and procedures (e.g. MedDRA).

Planning data checks

Once the requirements for an acceptable database have been defined, how should we plan to achieve this? A number of different approaches may be planned:

- Source data verification is an essential procedure for checking the accuracy of recording certain data. As the name implies, this involves the manual checking by the study monitor of the information recorded in the case report form, and subsequently in the database, with source documents stored by the investigator at the centre. Wherever possible this should be planned in advance to decide which variables are to be verified and for how many patient visits; 100% source data verification is often impractical.

- Pre-specified feasibility checks can be applied to certain variables at data entry such as checking that a value is within a plausible range or is one of a number of possible alternatives; this may be the actual recorded value or the value of a variable derived from this. It is advisable that this should all be carried out using validated programming steps specified at the planning stage. These checks may be automated to occur every time certain data points are entered into the system.

- Internal consistency of the database will need to be checked after the initial data entry has been completed as variables from different sections of the case report form may need to be compared. Where possible, such checks should be pre-specified and carried out using validated computer programmes. These checks are often automated.

- Checking for important missing data throughout the database should also be planned where possible. At the planning stage it may be recognized that data for certain variables will be incomplete and this will be handled by algorithms in the statistical programming; however, this does not reduce the importance of aiming to record complete data wherever possible.

Ideally, all specifications of the checking detailed in 'Planning data checks' would be considered at the planning stage and any changes made to the specification would be carefully described and recorded. Although it is sometimes necessary to make certain changes to the specification, these should be kept to a minimum.

Within trial data management

Overview

It is recommended that data be checked, queried, and corrected while the trial is being conducted. It is considerably easier to investigate potential errors in the database as soon as possible after the data have been collected. Therefore, whether paper collection or electronic data capture is used this requires data to be entered into the database with minimum delay. Data entry and management should be an ongoing exercise, which should only rarely be left until the completion of the actual conduct of the study. If data are queried promptly, problems can often be resolved quickly and easily. Therefore, regular checking of the database is essential.

Quality control of data entry

When data are entered from paper case report forms it is important to check the quality of the data entry to ensure that the information in the database agrees with what is recorded on the form. The data entry error rate may be considerably reduced by using double data entry where the same information is entered twice and then compared for inconsistencies. However, as this requires double the resource, single data entry is often preferred. In this case a planned procedure is necessary whereby a chosen percentage of the case report forms are compared with the data entered into the database. A high number of errors would prompt a larger sample to be checked or the data should be entered again in full.

Corrections to database

The regular examination of the database will identify a number of data points that require further investigation. Although it may sometimes appear to be obvious what the problem is, perhaps a decimal point incorrectly placed, the measurement in the wrong unit or even the components of a date in the wrong format, the data managers, programmers or statisticians should not make corrections to the database without the agreement of the relevant investigator. Therefore, a data query should be raised and documented together with any change that is made to the database. It is vital that all changes are tracked and clearly documented in order to maintain the integrity of the data. Any corrections made to the database without a clear paper trail or electronic record could create suspicion that the data have been manipulated and reduces confidence in the quality of the trial.

Completing the coding of data

In order to simplify the terminology used to describe medical conditions, and therapies and procedure used to treat them, it is common practice to use a recognized coding system or dictionary such as WHO drug for medications and MedDRA for medical conditions and procedures. Although an auto-encoder will automatically assign codes to a large percentage of the data, some free text will require manual coding by an experienced coder. Therefore it will be necessary to confirm the consistency of manual coding before the database is finally locked.

Regular examination of the database

The checking and validation of the database should be carefully planned in advance of study initiation. Some steps such as feasibility checks at data entry and source data verification will be an ongoing process. However, it is strongly recommended that other investigations such as consistency checks and identification of important missing data should be carried out at regular intervals usually based on the number of patient-visits available or the percentage of completed patients with all data entered into the database (e.g. 25%, 50%, 75%, and 100%). During the data review meeting held toward the end of the study it is often advisable to conduct a 'dry run' of the completed statistical analysis and reporting programmes which will be used to produce the tables, figures, and listings for the study report, as well as the analysis of the data. This will find any major problems with the data which have not yet been identified. It is important that this should not be carried out on unblinded data, but using a method of assigning patients to treatment groups using dummy randomization codes.

Locking and unlocking the database

- When all data have been carefully checked, all codes have been assigned and all outstanding queries are resolved, the study team should agree that the database is adequate for reporting and analysis.
- At this point the database is documented as being 'final' (often referred to as being 'locked' electronically) after which the randomization codes may be broken and the data made available to the statistician and statistical programmer.
- Occasionally it may be found that there is an important problem in the database which must be resolved in which case the database should be unlocked to correct this error. This can usually be avoided by proper planning and conducting the other checks described here, including a dry run of the programmes before the database is locked as described earlier.
- Unlocking the database is a very serious step and should only be considered if it is absolutely essential to make corrections. All changes made while the database is unlocked should be described and justified in the study report to maintain the integrity of the database. Following corrections the database should be locked again as quickly as possible.

Chapter 6.1

Pharmacovigilance

Pharmacovigilance

Pharmacovigilance is the science and activities relating to the detection, assessment, understanding, and prevention of adverse effects or any other drug-related problems.

Terminology

- An adverse event (AE) is any untoward medical occurrence in a patient or clinical investigation subject administered a pharmaceutical product and which does not necessarily have to have a causal relationship with this treatment.
- An adverse drug reaction (ADR) covers noxious and unintended effects resulting not only from the authorized use of a medicinal product at normal doses, but also from medication errors and uses outside the terms of the marketing authorization, including the misuse and abuse of the medicinal product.

There is at least a reasonable possibility of there being a causal relationship between a medicinal product and an adverse event.

There are four broad mechanisms for ADR which include exaggerated therapeutic response at the target site, pharmacological effect at another unintended site, additional secondary pharmacological actions, and immunological responses. ADR may be classified according to the A–E Classification or the DoTS categories:

A–E Classification

- Type A (Augmented pharmacological effects, common, predictable and dose related), e.g. bleeding with warfarin.
- Type B (Bizarre, not predictable from known pharmacology, not dose related, uncommon), e.g. anaphylaxis with penicillin.
- Type C (Chronic effects), e.g. lymphoma risk with ciclosporin.
- Type D (Delayed effects), e.g. tardive dyskinesia with neuroleptics.
- Type E (End of treatment effects), e.g. benzodiazepine withdrawal.

DoTS clinical pharmacology classification

- Dose (toxic, collateral or hypersusceptibility).
- Time (independent or dependent).
- Susceptibility (age, gender, ethnic origin, genetic or disease).
- Serious adverse event (SAE); a case is considered serious if it:
  - Resulted in a fatal outcome or is life threatening.
  - Led to hospitalization or prolonged hospitalization.
  - Led to persistent or significant disability.
  - Resulted in a congenital abnormality.
  - Is considered medically significant for other reasons.
- Unexpected adverse drug reaction is an adverse reaction, the nature or severity of which is not consistent with the applicable product information (investigator's brochure for investigational medicinal product or Summary of Product Characteristics for authorized product). Suspected unexpected serious adverse event (SUSAE) is a

serious adverse event that the nature, severity, specificity, or outcome is not consistent with the product information.

- EudraVigilance database is a data processing network and management system for reporting and evaluating suspected adverse reactions during the development and following the marketing authorization of medicinal products in the European Union.
- Post-authorization safety study (PASS): any study relating to an authorized medicinal product conducted with the aim of identifying, characterizing or quantifying a safety hazard, confirming the safety profile of the medicinal product, or of measuring the effectiveness of risk management measures.
- Post-authorization efficacy study (PAES): any study relating to an authorized medicinal product conducted where concerns relating to some aspects of the efficacy of the medicinal product are identified and can be resolved only after the medicinal product has been marketed.
- Risk management system: a set of pharmacovigilance activities and interventions designed to identify, characterize, prevent, or minimize risks relating to a medicinal product, including the assessment of the effectiveness of those activities and interventions. Risk management plan: a detailed description of the risk management system.
- Pharmacovigilance system master file: a detailed description of the pharmacovigilance system used by the marketing authorization holder with respect to one or more authorized medicinal products.
- Pharmacovigilance system: a system used by the marketing authorization holder and by member states to fulfil the tasks and responsibilities listed in Title IX and designed to monitor the safety of authorized medicinal products and detect any change to their risk–benefit balance.

Further reading

Directive 2010/84/EU. Available at: ℘ http://eudravigilance.ema.europa.eu/human/index.asp

Key pharmacovigilance regulations in the EU

Overview

EU legislation defines the roles and responsibilities of the key organizations involved in pharmacovigilance, in particular the pharmaceutical industry and regulatory authorities. The regulations apply to all MAs licensed (whether branded or generic, conventional, or herbal); however, they do not apply to homeopathic products (which are subject to a simplified registration procedure).

Key legislation and guidelines

The key pharmacovigilance legislation is Regulation (EU) No. 1235/2010 (amending, as regards pharmacovigilance of medicinal products for human use, Regulation (EC) No. 726/2004) and Directive 2010/84/EU (amending, as regards pharmacovigilance, Directive 2001/83/EC) which became applicable in July 2012. Detailed interpretation of the legislation is contained within the Good Pharmacovigilance Practices modules.

Organization of pharmacovigilance regulation in the EU

Effective pharmacovigilance relies on:
- Co-operation between national competent authorities (NCAs).
- Co-ordination provided by the European Medicines Agency (EMA).
- Compliance of MAHs (pharmaceutical companies) with the requirements of the legislation.

Pharmacovigilance risk assessment

The new legislation has created the Pharmacovigilance Risk Assessment Committee (PRAC), which has the primary responsibility for EU regulatory pharmacovigilance work. PRAC may issue opinions on any type of pharmacovigilance procedure (e.g. signals, RMP, PSURs, renewals, and safety referrals). PRAC opinions that involve centrally authorized products are routed to the EMA's Committee on Medicinal Products for Human Use (CHMP) for further consideration, while those for other products are routed through the Co-ordination Group for Mutual Recognition and Decentralized Procedures (human) (CMD(h)).

Key requirements of the regulations

Obligations placed upon MAHs and regulatory authorities are set out in the Good pharmacovigilance practice modules (See Chapter 6.3).

Pharmacovigilance inspections

Article 111 of Directive 2001/83/EC relates to the operation of pharmacovigilance inspections on MAHs in the EU. Inspections may be routine or targeted because of specific concerns. Inspection findings are categorized as 'critical', 'major' or 'minor'. MAHs are required to respond to the findings and initiate corrective or preventative measures within set timeframes. Identification of inadequate systems may lead to actions including re-inspections, warnings, and potentially fines or criminal proceedings.

Amendments to EU pharmacovigilance legislation (2012)

The pharmacovigilance legislation has resulted in key changes, which came into effect in July 2012.
- Establishment of a dedicated new committee, PRAC, which replaced the former Pharmacovigilance Working Party.
- Greater powers in relation to requesting and enforcing RMPs.
- Greater emphasis on monitoring new products and fewer requirements (e.g. PSURs) for well-established products.
- Streamlining of procedures, and greater transparency including web-portals for accessing data.

Further reading

EC Public Health Latest updates. Available at: ℞ http://ec.europa.eu/enterprise/sectors/pharmaceuticals/documents/eudralex/vol-9/index_en.htm

Good pharmacovigilance practices

Good pharmacovigilance practices (GVP)

Good pharmacovigilance practices (GVP) are guidelines drawn up to facilitate the performance of pharmacovigilance in the European Union (EU). The guidelines replace Volume 9A of the *Rules Governing Medicinal Products in the EU*. The GVP modules:
- Apply to MAHs and regulatory authorities.
- They cover centrally authorized medicinal products and medicines authorized at a national level.
- Each module presents one major pharmacovigilance process, divided into 3 sections; A, B, and C.
- Section A provides legal, technical, and scientific context.
- Section B gives guidance and reflects on scientific and regulatory approaches, formats, and standards agreed internationally.
- Section C covers the specifics of applying the approaches, formats and standards in the EU.
- There are 16 GVP modules covering major pharmacovigilance processes.
- The full set of modules is scheduled to be available during 2013 (some are currently under development as of late 2012).

Good pharmacovigilance practice modules (as of 2012)

- I: Pharmacovigilance systems and their quality systems.
- II: Pharmacovigilance system master file.
- III: Pharmacovigilance inspections.
- IV: Pharmacovigilance audits.
- V: Risk management systems.
- VI: Management and reporting of adverse reactions to medicinal products.
- VII: Periodic safety update report.
- VIII plus Annex: Post-authorization safety studies.
- IX: Signal management.
- X: Additional monitoring.
- XI: Public participation in pharmacovigilance.
- XII: Continuous pharmacovigilance, ongoing benefit–risk evaluation, regulatory action and planning of public communication.
- XIII: Incident management—incident management is no longer under development. All topics originally intended to be covered in this module are now to be included in module XII.

- XIV: International cooperation.
- XV: Safety communication.
- XVI: Risk-minimization measures: selection of tools and effectiveness indicators.

Further reading

EudraLex (2006). *Pharmacovigilance for Medicinal Products for Human Use.*
⅏ http://www.ema.europa.eu/ema/index.jsp?curl=pages/regulation/document_listing/document_listing_000345.jsp&mid=WC0b01ac058058f32c#section2

Periodic safety update reports

Overview

Periodic safety update reports (PSURs) are pharmacovigilance documents intended to provide an evaluation of the risk–benefit balance of a medicinal product for submission by MAHs at defined time points during the post-authorization phase. At these times, MAHs are expected to provide succinct summary information together with a critical evaluation of the risk–benefit balance of the product in the light of new or changing information. This evaluation should ascertain whether further investigations need to be carried out and whether changes should be made to the marketing authorization and the product information.

Regulatory requirements

As a result of the implementation of the new pharmacovigilance legislation, PSUR reporting is no longer required for all medicinal products. Certain products authorized under certain legal basis are exempt (Article 10.1 generic, Article 10a Well-established use, Article 14 Homeopathic medicine and Article 16a Traditional herbal medicine). However, PSURs may be requested on safety grounds for these products. The submission frequency of PSURs is decided on a risk-based approach, and the EMA publishes reference dates for PSUR as the EURD list.

The current situation for periodic safety reports on marketed drugs is different in the other 2 ICH regions. For example:

- The US FDA generally requires NDA periodic reports quarterly during the first 3yrs after the medicine is approved, and annual reports thereafter.
- In Japan, the authorities require a survey on a cohort of a few thousand patients established by a certain number of identified institutions during the 6yrs following approval, with systematic information reported annually on this cohort. Regarding other post-approval experience, adverse reactions that are non-serious, but both mild in severity and unlabelled, must be reported every 6mths for 3yrs and annually thereafter.

The content and format of a PSUR is specified in guidelines such as GVP Module VII and the ICH, which aims to harmonize global regulatory requirements:

- Introduction to the product.
- Worldwide approval status.
- Update on regulatory agency or pharmaceutical company actions taken for safety reasons.
- Changes to reference safety information.
- Data on patient exposure derived from an estimate of the number of patients exposed, along with the method used to calculate the estimate.
- Individual case histories.
- Discussion of company-sponsored and other studies yielding relevant safety information.

- Other information (efficacy-related information representing a significant hazard to the treated population and important late-breaking information).
- Overall safety evaluation, with specific highlighting/evaluation of:
  - Change in characteristics of listed reactions.
  - Serious unlisted reactions, placing cumulative reports into perspective.
  - Non-serious unlisted reactions.
  - Increased reporting frequency of listed reactions.
  - Any new safety issue (or lack of significant new information) regarding:
    - drug interactions;
    - experience with overdose, deliberate or accidental, and its treatment;
    - drug abuse or misuse;
    - positive or negative experiences during pregnancy or lactation;
    - experience in special patient groups (e.g. children, elderly, organ impaired);
    - effects of long-term treatment.

Conclusion

The PSUR can be an important source for the identification of new safety signals, a means of determining changes in the risk–benefit profile, an effective means of risk communication to regulatory authorities and an indicator for the need for risk management initiatives, as well as a tracking mechanism monitoring the effectiveness of such initiatives.

Further reading

ICH Topic E2C(R1). Clinical Safety Data Management: Periodic Safety Update Reports for Marketed Drugs. CPMP/ICH/288/95. Available at: ℘ http://www.ema.europa.eu/docs/en_GB/document_library/Scientific_guideline/2009/09/WC500002780.pdf

Good Pharmacovigilance Practices Module VII. Available at: ℘ http://www.ema.europa.eu/ema/index.jsp?curl=pages/news_and_events/news/2012/09/news_detail_001616.jsp&mid=WC0b01ac058004d5c1

Chapter 6.5

Benefit–risk assessment

Benefit–risk assessment

Benefit–risk assessment is the process by which the benefits (positive effects) and risks (probability of an adverse outcome) of a medicinal product are assessed and balanced to ensure that the adverse consequences of a medicine do not exceed the benefits (see Fig. 6.5.1). The process of balancing benefits and risks is a judgement one. There is no established mathematical method that simply combines benefit and risk data, permitting quantitative comparisons for decision making purposes.

Benefit–risk assessment is a continuous process, using a variety of sources of information and the assessment can only be as good as the quality of the underlying data. Benefit–risk evaluation should always be conducted relative to a suitable comparator therapy or to no therapy. The evaluation should include not just the effect of a new safety concern on the benefit–risk relationship, but should include a re-examination of the entire safety profile or at least the most important adverse drug reactions relative to other therapies. For the evaluation, the following concepts apply:

- The speed and intensity with which a benefit–risk evaluation is conducted is dependent on the medical seriousness of a suspected ADR.
- Consider the indication, whether there is an unmet clinical need and the performance of the drug under real conditions of use.
- Acceptable risk to whom? The acceptability of risk will be higher for life-threatening conditions.
- Take into account the strength of evidence and limitations of the data, all benefit–risk assessments are made in the face of uncertainty
- How could the interpretation change with the perceptions of different stakeholders (patients, healthcare professionals, pharmaceutical industry, regulatory authorities)?
- A MAH should immediately inform the CA of any new information that might influence the evaluation of the benefit–risk of a medicinal product.

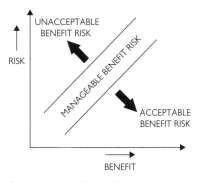

Fig. 6.5.1 Manageable benefit–risk.

Content of the benefit–risk evaluation report

The benefit–risk evaluation report should comprise an introduction, a benefit evaluation, a risk evaluation, a benefit–risk evaluation, options analysis, and decisions section:

- The introduction section should cover the drug specification, indication, disease context and the description of the suspected or established safety problem.
- The benefit evaluation describes the natural history of the target disease, the purpose of the treatment, the summary of efficacy and the tolerability compared with other existing therapies.
- The risk evaluation should cover the weight of evidence for suspected risk, analysis of the data, probable and possible explanations, preventability, predictability and reversibility, relationship with other alternative therapies/no therapy, and the review of the complete safety profile of the drug.
- The key section is the benefit–risk evaluation, which should pull together all the important elements of the assessment and summarize the benefits (purpose and effectiveness of treatment), summarize the principal risks (seriousness, severity, duration, and incidence), summarize the uncertainties and conclude with a benefit–risk relationship summary. The options analysis should consider what the most appropriate actions are. Here, the pros, cons, and consequences of each action are described and debated in an impact analysis. The actions may include:
- Maintaining the status quo.
- Watch and wait.
- Intensive additional gathering of data.
- Modifications to the use of the product or product literature.
- Restriction of product availability.
- Suspension.
- Withdrawal.
- Communication to the medical profession and or public.

Deciding on the appropriate course of action to take subsequent to a benefit–risk evaluation requires good decision-making practices and processes. There are three broad principles for decision-making—objectivity, equity, and accountability, and the basis and rationale of the decisions should be transparent. The outcome of the decision-making process should determining the actions to be taken, who should take them and the order and method of taking action. Drug safety communication should be accurate, balanced, open, understandable and targeted.

PROTECT EU project

There are a number of initiatives ongoing which aim to improve the process of benefit–risk evaluation. One such example is the Innovative Medicines Initiative PROTECT project which aims to improve scientific methods and strengthen the monitoring of the benefit–risk of medicines in Europe. The goal is to develop innovative methods which enhance early detection and assessment of ADRs from different data sources and to enable the integration and presentation of the data for continuous bene-fit–risk assessment/monitoring.

Further reading

CIOMS Working Group IV. Benefit-risk balance for marketed drugs: evaluating safety signals. Available at: ℜ http://www.cioms.ch/publications/g4-benefit-risk.pdf

IMI. Innovative Medicines Initiative. Available at: ℜ http://www.imi.europa.eu/

Pharmacoepidemiological safety data

Pharmacoepidemiology

Pharmacoepidemiology can be defined as the application of epidemiological methods to the study of the use, effectiveness, and safety of medicinal products. Pharmacoepidemiological studies aim to fill in the unknown, investigating under-represented groups, longer drug exposure, or safety signals. Such studies are largely based on observational data and they focus on measuring potential harms and safety in the real life post-marketing setting. Pharmacoepidemiology may provide evidence of association or no association, and four possible explanations for a positive association should be considered—causal effect, chance, bias, or confounding. Pharmacoepidemiological can be performed using a variety of data sources and methodologies (ICH E2E).

Spontaneous report

A spontaneous report is an unsolicited communication by healthcare professionals or consumers to a company, regulatory authority, or other organization that describes one or more ADRs in a patient who was given one or more medicinal products, and that does not derive from a study or any organized data collection scheme.

Cohort study

In a cohort study, users of a drug are identified and followed up to determine what events or ADRs occur. Typically, a cohort study will measure absolute and relative risks, and the approach is suited to the assessment of rare exposures.

Case control

In a case control study, cases of the reaction/event are identified and the use of the drug of interest is compared with controls without the reaction. A case control will measure an odds ratio and the approach is suited to the assessment of rare outcomes.

Registries

Registries consist of a list of patients with the same characteristics, such as a specific disease or drug exposure. Registries collect individual patient data, and the data is particularly useful for studying long-term effects, rare diseases, and rare exposures.

Drug utilization studies (DUS)

DUS investigate how a drug is marketed, prescribed and used in a specific population (e.g. elderly, children, or patients with hepatic or renal impairment). The studies explore the determinants of drug use, reasons for variation in drug use, assess the appropriateness of prescribing, misuse and off label use and determine the medical, social, and economic consequences.

Prescription event monitoring (PEM)

PEM is an intensive monitoring scheme that aims to monitor all new products expected to be used widely by general practitioners (GP). Patients taking specific medicines are identified and a questionnaire is sent to their GP at pre-specified intervals in order to obtain outcome information. In the UK, the scheme is co-ordinated by the Drug Safety Research Unit (DSRU). Event rates can be compared during and after exposure, and over time.

The European Network of Centres for Pharmacoepidemiology and Pharmacovigilance (ENCePP)

The ENCePP project is led by the EMA, with a goal to strengthen post-authorization monitoring of medicinal products by conducting multi-centre independent studies that focus on benefit risk and safety. The ENCePP has produced a Code of Conduct for scientific independence and transparency in the conduct of pharmacoepidemiological and pharmacovigilance studies. The use of the Code is voluntary, but it is mandatory if a study is to be awarded the title of ENCePP study. By agreeing to follow the Code, investigators and study funders commit to adhere to the following general principles:

- The primary purpose of a study shall be to generate data of potential scientific or public health importance, and not to promote the sale of a medicinal product.
- The design of the research shall not be aimed towards producing a pre-specified result.
- A contract shall be concluded between the (primary) lead investigator or the co-ordinating study entity and the study funder clearly defining the research assignment and addressing in sufficient detail critical areas of their interaction, remuneration, protocol agreement, analysis of results, and publication of results.
- Remuneration shall only be granted as specified in the research contract and shall not depend on the study results.
- The results of a study shall always be published, preferably in a peer-reviewed journal, or made available for public scrutiny within an acceptable time frame, regardless of the (positive or negative) results and the statistical significance.
- Relevant information on the research process and results shall be made publicly available or on request as specified in the Code.

Further reading

ICH. Pharmacovigilance planning. Available at: ℘ http://www.ich.org/fileadmin/Public_Web_Site/ICH_Products/Guidelines/Efficacy/E2E/Step4/E2E_Guideline.pdf
Drug Safety Research Unit. Available at: ℘ http://www.dsru.org/
ENCePP. Available at: ℘ http://www.encepp.eu/

Product suspension and withdrawal and defective medicines

Product suspension and withdrawal

Following the assessment of a safety concern, the benefit–risk evaluation should determine the appropriate measures to be taken to minimize the risks to public health. In extreme cases, where the benefit risk is considered to no longer be positive, risk minimization actions may include product suspension or withdrawal from the market. Article 116 and 117 of Directive 2001/83/EC specifies under what circumstances medicinal products may be suspended or withdrawn. According to Article 116 'the competent authorities shall suspend, revoke, withdraw or vary a marketing authorization if the view is taken that the product is harmful under normal conditions of use, or that it lacks therapeutic efficacy, or that the risk–benefit balance is not positive under the normal conditions of use, or that its qualitative and quantitative composition is not as declared.' Furthermore, Article 117 states that member states shall take all appropriate steps to ensure that the supply of the medicinal product is prohibited.

Temporary suspension of a marketed product may be considered when the magnitude of a safety problem is still to be fully determined. The suspension may be short- or long-term, and if the safety problem is resolved, the manufacturer may resume marketing without having to submit a new drug application. Although withdrawal is probably the least desirable option for either the regulatory agency or the manufacture, it may be essential if the risks of using a medicinal product outweigh the beneficial effects.

The decision to withdraw a product should be considered relative to the indication, available alternative treatments, and following attempts to minimize the risks and maximize the benefits. Withdrawal from the market is particularly problematic for chronic use products and it may be possible for some patients to continue using a product on a compassionate use basis. For newly-identified risks that are considered to be serious and an imminent hazard to patients, the regulator may consider it necessary to alert healthcare professionals and the public and to initiate an immediate recall. In such circumstances the following items should be considered:

• How severe would be the harm that the drug might cause pending the completion of a customary review and procedure for its withdrawal or restriction.
• How likely is the drug to cause such harm to users during a less immediate administrative process.
• What risk would immediate withdrawal pose to current users, given the availability of other therapies and the need for patients to adjust to them.
• Are there other approaches to protecting public health.
• What is the best judgement, given the information available at the time, of the likelihood that the drug will be withdrawn on the completion of the more customary administrative process.

Defective medicines

In clinical practice it may be difficult to differentiate between adverse drug reactions and defective medicinal products, e.g. an increase in the incidence of ADRs, which appear to be associated with one batch of product. A defective medicine is one whose quality does not conform to the requirements of its marketing authorization or specification. In the UK, the MHRA's Defective Medicines Report Centre (DMRC) aims to minimize the hazards arising from the distribution of defective medicinal products by providing an emergency assessment and communication system between manufactures, distributors, regulatory authorities, and end users. If it is determined that the withdrawal of the product is necessary, it is the MAHs responsibility to recall the defective product. However, depending on the scale of problem and the nature of the risk, the DMRC may issue a drug alert to supplement any action taken by the MAH.

Levels of risk
- *Class 1:* the defect presents a life-threatening or serious risk to health. The recall should generally be at the patient level.
- *Class 2:* the defect may cause mistreatment or harm to the patient, but is not life threatening or serious. Patient level recalls are rarely required.
- *Class 3:* the defect is unlikely to cause harm to the patient, and the recall is carried out for other reasons, such as non-compliance with the marketing authorization or specification.
- *Class 4:* there is no threat to patients or no serious defect likely to impair the product use or efficacy.

Further reading
CIOMS. Available at: ℬ www.cioms.ch
MHRA. Defective Medicines Report Centre. Available at: ℬ http://www.mhra.gov.uk/Safetyinformation/
    Howwemonitorthesafetyofproducts/Medicines/DefectiveMedicinesReportCentre/CON019692

Chapter 6.8

Safety signal

Safety signal

The World Health Organization (WHO) defines a signal as 'reported information on a possible causal relationship between an adverse event and a drug, the relationship being unknown or incompletely documented previously.' The term also applies when there is new evidence that a known hazard may be quantitatively (change in frequency) or qualitatively (change in seriousness) different from what was previously known. Therefore, a safety signal is an early marker of a potential hazard, which arouses suspicion and stimulates further investigation. For signal detection, usually more than one report is required, although this depends upon the seriousness of the event and the quality of the information.

Signal detection

Very common, common, and uncommon ADRs may be detected during the clinical development programme, but rare and very rare ADR are generally only detected by market surveillance. The objective of signal detection is to identify such rare ADR and to identify high risk groups of patients. Signals may be generated by a number of different data gathering methods, including cohort studies, published case reports, post-marketing clinical studies, and spontaneous reporting.

Data mining is an analysis by automatic or semi-automatic means of large quantities of raw data in order to extract previously unknown relationships or patterns. Such computerized methods involve statistical measures of disproportionality (whether or not more reports have been received than might have been expected as background noise) and include proportional reporting ratio (PRR), reporting odds ratio (ROR), information component (IC) and multi-item Gamma-Poisson Shrinker (MGPS).

In the context of spontaneous reporting, a signal is normally a series of similar cases reported in relation to a particular drug and three cases are generally considered to be adequate. However, for certain types of event that are particularly important and that are strongly likely to be drug-related (e.g. anaphylaxis), a single case may be sufficient to raise a signal.

Signal prioritization

Signal prioritization includes triage and impact analysis. The most important features of a case are assessed rapidly during triage in order to determine the urgency for further evaluation and assessment relative to other cases. Impact analysis is a quantitative method that involves calculating two scores, used to determine the overall priority of the case.

- The evidence score, based on the degree of disproportionality, strength of evidence and plausibility.
- The public health score, based on the numbers of reported cases in a year, expected health consequences and reporting rate in relation to the level of drug exposure.

The overall categories derived from these scores are classed as high priority, need to gather more information, low priority, and no action.

Signal clarification and evaluation

Deciding on whether or not a drug was responsible for an adverse event is rarely straight forward and requires judgement. In making such judgements, the Bradford–Hill criteria (strength, consistency, specificity, temporality, biological gradient, plausibility, coherence, experimental evidence) provide a framework for linking a new signal with causality. The more criteria that are met, the more likely an association is causal:
- Are there previous conclusive reports on this reaction?
- Did the adverse event appear after the suspected drug was administered?
- Did the adverse event improve when the drug was discontinued?
- Did the adverse event reappear if the drug was re-administered?
- Are there alternative causes?
- Did the reaction occur with placebo?
- Was the drug detected in the blood?
- Was the reaction more severe when the dose was increased or less severe when the dose was decreased?
- Did the patient have a similar reaction to the same or similar drug in any previous exposure?
- Was the adverse event confirmed by any objective means?
- Does the balance of evidence support cause and effect?

Outcome

The likelihood that a signal is caused by the drug is categorized as; probable/likely (balance of information supports causation), possible (some information is in favour of causation), unlikely (balance of information does not support causation), and unassessable (key information is missing). The outcome of a signal will be based on the benefit–risk profile and what are the likely clinical implications (severity, fatal, or life-threatening). The outcomes following a signal evaluation include:
- No action/unconfirmed.
- Intensive monitoring/further study.
- Include in PSUR.
- Refer to safety committee to change label.
- Notify regulatory authorities and senior management.
- Update the RMP and consider additional risk minimization measures.

Further reading

CIOMS. Available at: ℘ http://www.cioms.ch/

Spontaneous reporting

Spontaneous reporting

Single case reports represent the most important source of information for raising safety suspicions and generating early safety signals in the post-marketing authorization setting. A spontaneous report is defined as an unsolicited communication by a healthcare professional or consumer to a company, regulatory authority, or other organization, which fulfils the following three conditions:
- It describes one or more suspected adverse reactions in a patient.
- The patient was given one or more medicinal products.
- It does not derive from a study or any organized data collection scheme.

The minimum criteria for reporting are:
- An identifiable patient.
- A suspected medicinal product.
- An identifiable reporting source.
- An event or outcome.

Spontaneous reporting relies heavily on the alertness of the prescribing clinician or other reporter, and on the quality of the operational system. Spontaneous reporting raises suspicions. Numerous reports linking rare exposures to rare outcomes may be sufficient to establish a strong association. However, data from spontaneous reporting alone is generally not sufficient to establish causality or estimate risk, and such passive surveillance should be complemented with more formal approaches for the characterization of potential hazards.

Benefits of spontaneous reporting
- Provides early warnings of previously unrecognized adverse drug reactions.
- Schemes are relatively inexpensive to run.
- Can be applied to all drugs.
- Potentially covers the whole population, providing safety signals in a continuous manner.
- Possible identification of predisposing risk factors.

Limitations of spontaneous reporting
- Schemes are susceptible to under reporting.
- Schemes are susceptible to over reporting (for drugs in the media spot light).
- Cannot normally calculate incidence as limited information on patient exposure.
- Reports are only observations of suspected association.
- Difficulty in recognizing previously unknown drug reactions.

Yellow Card Scheme

The Yellow Card Scheme is the UK's spontaneous reporting scheme. It is administered by the MHRA and the CHM, with the support of five Yellow Card Centres. The scheme was established in 1964 following the Thalidomide tragedy, which highlighted the need for routine monitoring of medicines.

The Yellow Card reporting scheme receives more than 20 000 suspected ADR reports per year from healthcare professionals (doctors, pharmacists, nurses) and patients. The reports are made on a voluntary basis, and cover both licensed and unlicensed medicines (and herbal preparations). Reports are entered onto the MHRA's database together with a unique identification number. The database facilitates the monitoring of ADRs and allows rapid analysis of spontaneous reports. A team of safety experts uses the data from the reports to assess the causal relationship between the drug and the reported reaction(s). Possible risk factors contributing to the occurrence of the reaction are also investigated, including analysis of relevant data from other sources.

The Yellow Card

- The Yellow Card contains the following sections:
  - The patient's details, the suspected drug(s).
  - The suspected reaction(s).
  - Drugs taken in the preceding 3 months and reporter's details.

Further reading

MHRA. The Yellow Card Sceme. Available at: ℰ http://yellowcard.mhra.gov.uk/the-yellow-card-scheme/

Chapter 6.10

Post-authorization safety studies

Overview

A post-authorization safety study (PASS) is any study relating to an author-ized medicinal product conducted with the aim of identifying, character-izing, or quantifying a safety hazard, confirming the safety profile of the medicinal product, or of measuring the effectiveness of risk management measures.

Post-authorization safety studies may be conducted for the purpose of identifying previously unrecognized safety concerns (hypothesis-generation), investigating potential and identified risks (hypothesis-testing in order to substantiate a causal association), or confirming the known safety profile of a medicinal product under normal conditions of use. They may also be conducted to quantify established adverse reactions and to identify risk factors.

Studies may be appropriate in the following situations:
- A medicine with a novel structure or mode of action.
- Uncertainty as to the safety profile.
- Better quantification of adverse events identified in clinical trials.
- To confirm or refute safety concerns.
- To evaluate the effectiveness of a risk management plan.
  A variety of designs may be appropriate, including:
- Observational cohort studies.
- Case-control studies.
- Registries.
- Clinical trials involving systematic allocation of treatment.

The MAH who initiates the study is responsible for its conduct and should meet the pharmacovigilance obligations regarding PASS. The QPPV or nominated person responsible for pharmacovigilance at national level should be involved in the review of the protocols.

The MAH proposing to perform a PASS should send the protocol to the CA of the MS(s) in whose territory the study is to be performed. Two different situations can be envisaged depending on whether or not the study has been requested by the CAs.

Studies requested by competent authorities

MAHs should provide a study progress report annually, or more fre-quently, as requested by the CAs (e.g. according to the RMP milestones) or on their own initiative. If the study is discontinued, a final report should also be submitted.

Studies performed at the MAHs initiative

- Progress and final reports should be included or updated in the corresponding PSUR and/or RMP. When a safety concern is raised, a report should be submitted immediately to the relevant CAs (including the EMA and (Co-) Rapporteur for centrally authorized products and the RMS for products authorized through the mutual recognition process.
- Post-authorization studies should not be planned or conducted for the purposes of promoting the use of medicinal products.

- Company sales and marketing representatives should not be involved in studies in such a way that it could be seen as a promotional exercise, such as in the recruitment of patients and physicians.

Further reading

GVP Module VIII. Available at: ℜ http://www.ema.europa.eu/ema/index.jsp?curl=pages/regulation/document_listing/document_listing_000345.jsp&mid=WC0b01ac058058f32c#section2

Dear Healthcare Professional communication

Overview

A Dear Healthcare Professional letter (DHPL) is a communication tool, which forms an important part of any risk mitigation strategy (known as a Risk Evaluation & Mitigation strategies (REMs) plan in the US) for a pharmaceutical product. Specific guidance exists around the reasons for issuing and construct for a DHPL issued by both the FDA and the EMEA.

Reasons for issuing a DHPL

The main reasons for issuing a DHPL are to do with availability of new safety data which significantly affects the risk–benefit balance for use of a particular medicine. Examples of events that have precipitated availability of new safety information over the past few years include large phase III studies, meta-analyses, and analyses of spontaneously reported adverse events in clinical practice.

Key components of a DHPL

Summary of new information

The DHPL should start with a summary of new information, which has become available, and draws some conclusions around this as to how the information could impact on the benefit risk for the particular agent concerned.

Advice on how the new information can impact on clinical practice

What changes to current use of the agent may be necessary? Examples:
• Patients who should now be ruled out for treatment.
• New tests which may be required prior to starting treatment.
• Monitoring required whilst on therapy.

What is the exact/proposed change in wording for the label?

This section of the letter would ordinarily contain a section of the label that pertains to the new information, any new testing required, and any new requirements for screening-out elements of the population who were previously applicable for the medicine.

Who is the country contact for further information?

What is the telephone number, email address, and physical address, and name of a key contact for the marketing authorization holder who can help with providing further information?

Further reading

FDA review process for DHPLs. Available at: ℘ http://www.fda.gov/downloads/AboutFDA/CentersOffices/CDER/ManualofPoliciesProcedures/ucm082012.pdf

GCP Module XV. Available at: ℘ http://www.ema.europa.eu/ema/index.jsp?curl=pages/regulation/document_listing/document_listing_000345.jsp&mid=WC0b01ac058058f32c#section2

Issues and crisis management

Overview

> *If you can keep your head when all about you*
> *Are losing theirs and blaming it on you;*
> *If you can trust yourself when all men doubt you*
> > Rudyard Kipling

Whilst an issue, when it arises, can seem like a disaster, anything can be sorted out with meticulous planning.

Defining the problem

Defining the nature of the problem is crucial and escalating appropriately. Early discussion centres on the evaluation of patient safety, necessity, and timelines to inform regulatory authorities, and a decision as to whether withdrawal of a marketed or investigational product is required.

Ideally, a summary is compiled defining the issue, consequences, and potential remediation plan. This is then presented to the chief medical officer for review/endorsement.

If there is deemed to be a significant patient safety issue, a need for withdrawal of investigational product or a marketed agent, or a significant new piece of data impacting on benefit risk, for example, a crisis can be declared.

In the event of a crisis, experts are recruited in managing functions which are significantly impacted by the event. During the crucial early period meetings daily or even twice daily may be indicated.

Typical members of the crisis team

- *Chair:* usually the chief medical officer or global head of safety.
- *Project physician:* lead physician responsible for the agent.
- *Project scientist:* scientist supporting the agent concerned.
- *Regulatory lead:* to advise on negotiations/liaison with the regulator.
- *Manufacturing lead:* to advise about remediation for manufacturing issues.
- *Logistics and supply chain:* advice on logistics of a product withdrawal.
- *Country medical heads where issue has occurred:* to advise on local market issues.
- *Media affairs:* to advise on communication issues with respect to the general public or financial media.

Closing the loop

Once the issue is resolved the crisis team should circle back to measure/
examine the time period for resolution, review any media reaction, any
regulatory response, and take any learnings forward to:
• Reduce the likelihood of a future crisis.
• Ensure that lessons are taken forward to manage a future event more
  efficiently.

Chapter 6.13

Adverse events in clinical trials

Adverse events

The objectives of collecting adverse events in clinical trials includes detecting and characterizing ADRs, investigating the relationship between dose and safety, protecting trial subjects from harm and fulfilling legal obligations. Accordingly, the Clinical Trials Directive 2001/20/EC states that a clinical trial may be initiated only if the Ethics Committee and/or competent authority comes to the conclusion that the anticipated therapeutic and public health benefits justify the risks and may be continued only if compliance with this requirement is permanently monitored. Therefore, it is crucial to have robust mechanisms in place to collect, verify, and report adverse events in clinical trials. Article 16 of the Directive describes the requirements for notification of adverse events:

• The investigator shall report all serious adverse events immediately to the sponsors except for those that the protocol or investigators brochure identifies as not requiring immediate reporting and the immediate report should be followed up by detailed written reports, identifying subjects by unique codes.
• Adverse events identified in the protocol as critical to safety evaluations shall be reported to the sponsor according to the reporting requirements and within the time periods specified in the protocol.

With regards to serious adverse events, the sponsor shall ensure that;

• All relevant information about suspected unexpected serious adverse reactions that are fatal or life-threatening is recorded and reported as soon as possible to competent authorities in all the MSs concerned and to the Ethics Committee, and in any case no later than 7 days. Relevant follow-up information should be subsequently communicated within an additional 8 days.
• All other suspected unexpected serious adverse reactions shall be reported to the competent authorities concerned and to the Ethics Committee as soon as possible, but within a maximum of 15 days of first knowledge by the sponsor.

Clinical trial design

The sponsor should anticipate findings and design trials according to all available safety data. The sponsor should consider:

• The preclinical data.
• The mechanism of action.
• The target disease and symptomology.
• Potential concomitant medication.
• Any known class effect.

All adverse events occurring in trial subjects after drug exposure should be systematically and proactively recorded on the case report form. Detailed guidance on the collection, verification, and presentation of adverse events in clinical trials is found in EC guidance ENTR/CT 3. This document covers the responsibilities of the investigator and sponsor, and describes best practice for the reporting of adverse reactions. Other important regulatory guidance documents include the ICH E2 series of Topics (A–F).

- Collected safety data should be thoroughly investigated and assessed against a background of ongoing benefit risk analysis.
- The sponsor should promptly notify the competent authorities if safety issues emerge that may impact on the study conduct or may alter the clinical trial authorization.
- The identification of a serious new hazard may lead to a trial being suspended or terminated.

Article 12 of Directive 2001/20/EC establishes that 'where a member state has objective grounds for considering that the conditions in the request for authorization referred to in Article 9(2) are no longer met or has information raising doubts about the safety or scientific validity of the clinical trial, it may suspend or prohibit the clinical trial and shall notify the sponsor thereof'.

Independent Data Monitoring Committee (IDMC)

The IDMC (also called the Data Safety Monitoring Board—DSMB) is a committee made up of impartial experts that periodically reviews and analyses data, normally during the course of large clinical trials. The objective of the committee is to assess at intervals the appropriateness of continuing a clinical trial based on accumulated data. Adverse events that are reported by trial investigators are complied and reviewed by the committee in order to ensure that trial subjects are not exposed to unnecessary risk. On safety grounds, the committee may recommend the sponsor modifies the trial protocol or terminates the trial.

Development safety update report (DSUR)

It is a requirement of EU Directive 2001/20/EC that competent authorities and ethics committees are provided with a safety report on an annual basis. The DSUR is intended to serve as an annual report and to be a common standard for periodic reporting on drugs under development, including marketed drugs that are undergoing further study (ICH E2F). The main objective of a DSUR is to present a comprehensive annual review and evaluation of safety information collected during the reporting period by:

- Examining whether the information obtained by the sponsor during the reporting period is in accord with previous knowledge.
- Describing new safety issues that could have an impact on the protection of clinical trial subjects.
- Summarizing the current understanding and management of identified and potential risks.

- Providing an update on the status of the clinical investigation or development programme and study results.

Further reading

ICH website. Available at: ℘ https://www.ich.org
EC Public Health. Medicinal products for human use. Available at: ℘ http://ec.europa.eu/health/human-use/clinical-trials/index_en.htm

Chapter 6.14

Risk management

Overview

For a new medicinal product, not all actual or potential risks will have been identified at the time of marketing authorization, and safety information may be relatively limited. This is due to many factors, but includes the small numbers of subjects entered into clinical trials, the restricted population in terms of age, gender, ethnicity, co-morbidity, co-medication, and conditions of use, and the relatively short duration of exposure and follow-up.

A risk management system is a set of pharmacovigilance activities and interventions designed to identify, characterize, prevent, or minimize risks relating to a medicinal product, including the assessment of the effectiveness of those activities and interventions. A risk management plan (RMP) is a detailed description of the risk management system.

The aim of a risk management system is to ensure that the benefits exceed the risks by the greatest possible margin, both for the individual patient and for the wider population. This can be achieved either by increasing the benefits or by reducing the risks. The management of a risk signal consists of four steps: risk detection, assessment, minimization, and communication.

European risk management plan

In Europe, the detailed description of the requirements for a risk management system can be found in the Good Pharmacovigilance Practice (GVP) Module V. RMPs are required for all new marketing authorization applications. Risk management consists of:

- Characterization of the safety profile of the medicinal product, including what is known and not known.
- Planning of pharmacovigilance activities to characterize risks and identify new risks and increase the knowledge in general about the safety profile of the medicinal product.
- Planning and implementation of risk minimization and mitigation and assessment of the effectiveness of these activities the risk–benefit balance, risks need to be understood in the context of benefit.

In relation to risk management of its medicinal products, an applicant/ MAH is responsible for:

- Ensuring that it constantly monitors the risks of its medicinal products in compliance with relevant legislation and reports the results of this, as required, to the appropriate competent authorities.
- Taking all appropriate actions to minimize the risks of the medicinal product and maximize the benefits, including ensuring the accuracy of all information produced by the company in relation to its medicinal products, and actively updating and promptly communicating it when new information becomes available.

Structure of the risk management plan

The RMP is a dynamic, stand-alone document which should be updated throughout the lifecycle of medicinal products. The RMP consists of seven parts. The EMA will make available on its website a template for the RMP (during 2013).
- Part I Product(s) overview.
- Part II Safety specification:
  - Module SI Epidemiology of the indication(s) and target population(s).
  - Module SII Non-clinical part of the safety specification.
  - Module SIII Clinical trial exposure.
  - Module SIV Populations not studied in clinical trials.
  - Module SV Post-authorization experience.
  - Module SVI Additional EU requirements for the safety specification.
  - Module SVII Identified and potential risks.
  - Module SVIII Summary of the safety concerns.
- Part III Pharmacovigilance plan.
- Part IV Plans for post-authorization efficacy studies.
- Part V Risk minimization measures (including evaluation of the effectiveness of risk minimization measures).
- Part VI Summary of the risk management plan.
- Part VII Annexes.

Objectives of a risk management plan

The RMP must contain the following elements which do the following:
- Identify or characterize the safety profile of the medicinal product(s) concerned.
- Indicate how to characterize further the safety profile of the medicinal product(s) concerned.
- Document measures to prevent or minimise the risks associated with the medicinal product including an assessment of the effectiveness of those interventions.
- Document post-authorization obligations that have been imposed as a condition of the marketing authorization.
- Describe what is known and not known about the safety profile of the concerned medicinal product(s).
- Indicate the level of certainty that efficacy shown in clinical trial populations will be seen when the medicine is used in the wider target populations seen in everyday medical practice and document the need for studies on efficacy in the post-authorization phase (also known as effectiveness studies).
- Include a description of how the effectiveness of risk minimization measures will be assessed.

Further reading

GVP Module VIII. Available at: http://www.ema.europa.eu/ema/index.jsp?curl=pages/regulation/document_listing/document_listing_000345.jsp&mid=WC0b01ac058058f32c#section2

Section 7

Healthcare marketplace

Marketing medicines: the drug lifecycle

Overview

Marketing of medicines is an essential activity, to inform healthcare professionals about new treatment options available and to enable them to provide the most appropriate treatment for their patients. It is also important to allow companies to gain adequate return on the significant research and development (R&D) investment within the period of patent protection and market exclusivity, so that they can continue to invest in new treatments.

The marketing mix

The major marketing management decisions can be classified in one of the following four categories:
- *Product:* the product is the medicine itself. It includes aspects such as efficacy, safety, mode of delivery, and other factors that may differentiate the product from competitors.
- *Price:* ensure good return on investment with premium price but get access via positive HTA or formulary inclusion.
- *Place (distribution):* target the correct customers. Try early adopters first.
- *Promotion:* key selling messages and value added services, including patient materials.

These variables are known as the marketing mix or the 4 P's of marketing. They are the variables that marketers can control in order to best satisfy customers in the target market. The marketing mix is portrayed in Fig. 7.1.1.

The marketing mix should be adapted to the challenges and opportunities at each stage of the lifecycle.

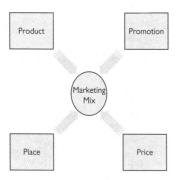

Fig. 7.1.1 The marketing mix.

The drug lifecycle

The marketing activities a company engages in depends on a number of factors. However, it is the lifecycle phase which will determine what strategies are implemented.

Fig. 7.1.2 illustrates the sales growth curve of a typical drug lifecycle. Irrespective of the actual sales that are eventually achieved, this typical lifecycle can be broken down into 4 main phases: Introduction, growth, maturity, and decline. It is the growth phase that offers pharmaceutical companies the greatest opportunities to influence their revenue prospects. The rate of growth in this phase determines the peak sales that can be achieved in the plateau phase and, therefore, a product's overall commercial potential.

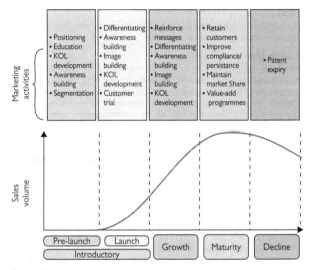

Fig. 7.1.2 Typical drug lifecycle curve.

Introductory phase

Pre-launch planning spans multiple years and involves the co-ordination of highly disparate activities. The marketing goals in this period include:

• *Leveraging thought leaders:* this will help you ensure messages are resonant with healthcare professionals and ensure that the target market is correctly identified and segmented. They can also advise on appropriate activities to educate the marketplace. This is particularly important for a new class of therapy.

- *Building awareness can be achieved through conference preference:* creating meaningful product differentiation. Differentiation goes beyond claims about efficacy and safety. It includes:
  - Added value to potential customers, ranging from patients to physicians to payers.
  - Rigorous scientific data.
  - Other services and products.
  - Convey how a treatment will fit into a clinical practice, which patients will benefit.
  - Identifying what reimbursement levels and formulary placement are appropriate from a payer perspective.
- *Market research:* in order to differentiate and deliver the value necessary for a successful launch, marketers have to understand market dynamics including patient flows and physician segments in the market.
- *Sales force buy in.*
- *Create initial positive experiences:* that builds market credibility, which allows marketing expansion over time.

Growth phase

This builds on a successful launch period. This is an important phase that requires significant sales force activity to reinforce the products key messages and build differentiation. It is important to ensure that compliance and persistence with treatment is supported to ensure stable sales. Programmes to achieve this may be considered. Disseminating positive clinical outcomes will build credibility and trust in the product and will drive further adoption by physicians, although leaders must continue to be leveraged to build awareness of the product and credibility in its offerings. During this phase, products become more profitable and companies form alliances, joint ventures, and take each other over. Advertising spend is high and focuses upon building a brand. Competitors are also attracted into the market with very similar offerings.

Maturity phase

In this phase, sales grow at a decreasing rate and then stabilize. The primary goal now is to protect market share. During this phase it is important to retain existing patients with compliance and persistence programmes. Efforts must also be made to retain existing prescribers. Investment in other value-add programmes may also be considered. It is likely that the market will be crowded with competitors so differentiation of the product remains important.

Decline phase

Following patent expiry, generic alternative may quickly enter the market. Usually there is disinvestment in the product at this stage.

The Foreign Corrupt Practices Act and UK Bribery Act

Overview

The Foreign Corrupt Practices Act (FCPA) is a US federal law enacted in 1977, prohibiting companies from paying bribes to foreign government officials and political figures. Companies violating this law by paying bribes are subject to criminal and civil actions, which can result in fines, suspension, and exclusion from government procurement contracts, while the employees and directors can be subject to prison sentences.

Principal provisions

The FCPA has two principal provisions—the anti-bribery prohibitions, and the books and records requirements:

- *Anti-bribery prohibitions:* the FCPA prohibits bribery of non-US government officials by US nationals. This prohibits providing anything of value to a government official to obtain or retain business. This includes travel, scholarships, and charitable contributions.
- *Books and records:* the FCPA also requires the maintenance of accurate books, records, and accounting controls. Companies must ensure compliance by foreign subsidiaries.

Reach of the foreign corrupt practices

The reach of the FCPA is broad and includes:

- US companies and its officers, directors, employees, and agents.
- US citizens and residents wherever located.
- Non-US subsidiaries of US companies.
- Anyone who commits a bribe within the US.
- Bribes by agents or third parties on your behalf, with your knowledge. (See Box 7.2.1 below for details).

Box 7.2.1 Third parties

- Agents.
- Consultants.
- Contractors.
- Brokers.
- Joint venture partners.
- Distributors.
- Licensees.

Knowledge means:

- Awareness of a 'high probability' that prohibited conduct will occur.
- Conscious disregard, willful blindness, or deliberate ignorance of prohibited conduct.

Risk areas

In the pharmaceutical industry there are a number of key risk areas. Interactions with healthcare professionals and government bodies is one of these and includes:
- Fees for speaking.
- Consulting or service arrangements.
- Clinical trials:
  - Pre- and post-market studies.
  - Conduct of the clinical trial.
- Compensation/fair market value.
- Gifts and hospitality.
- Educational grants and charitable donation.

It is therefore, important that companies conduct an appropriate level of due diligence in connection with transactions in order to:
- Identify and mitigate risk of violations of the FCPA.
- Avoid involvement in transactions that might expose the company to unmanageable risk.
- Demonstrate that the company acted responsibly in the event issues arise later.

Companies should conduct due diligence before entering into relationships with consultants, agents, distributors, and other third parties. The four principles that should be followed are shown in Table 7.2.1.

Table 7.2.1 Principles of working with third parties

Separation	Transparency	Equivalence	Documentation
• A clear separation should exist between benefit given and decision to purchase/ prescribe product	• Benefits should be disclosed	• Any payment for services should not exceed fair market value for that service	• All interaction should have clear and robust documentation

UK Bribery Act

Recently, the United Kingdom passed its own version of the FCPA, the UK Bribery Act, which is stricter and more punitive than the FCPA. The main provisions of the UKBA 2010 came into force in July 2011.

The Bribery Act creates the following four offences:

- *Active bribery:* promising or giving a financial or other advantage.
- *Passive bribery:* agreeing to receive or accepting a financial or other advantage.
- Bribery of foreign public officials.
- The failure of commercial organizations to prevent bribery by an associated person.

The Bribery Act also covers bribes by agents or third parties on your behalf, with or without your knowledge and applies to UK citizens, residents, and companies established under UK law. In addition, non-UK companies can be held liable for a failure to prevent bribery if they do business in the UK.

The scope of the law is extra-territorial. Under the Bribery Act, a relevant person or company can be prosecuted for the above crimes if the crimes are committed abroad.

Sanctions increase under the Bribery Act to a maximum of 10 years imprisonment and an unlimited fine.

Product lifecycle management

Overview

Traditionalists might think of lifecycle management as just managing the tail, the time for switch away from active promotion, timing of any partnership with a generic company, or the moment for POM to P switch, but actually lifecycle management should begin in phase II.

Pre-phase III

Early on, preferably when the results from phase IIa are available, a visioning process is essential. This involves prediction of the likely magnitude of clinical effect, assessment of likely competitors at launch, price achievable, physician, patient, and payer attitudes in the current timeframe, and the desired attitudes to prescribing at time of launch.

Ideally, this visioning process should identify a so-called 'lead indication,' where greatest unmet need for patients and likely most rapid uptake in prescribing has been identified. It should also identify follow on indications, which may be in complementary patient populations, or a different disease area altogether.

The process is revisited at the end of phase IIb, at which stage more clinical data has become available, coupled with the results of detailed payer research, which drives design of endpoints in the phase III programme, targeted at meeting reimbursement needs.

Post-phase III

Negotiations about price/access and any volume cap occur according to local in country regulations; these drive either confirmation or revision of initial assumptions about annual sales, and a potential IIIb/IV programme to enhance clinical knowledge about the attributes of the agent.

Filings for expansion of the indication for an existing disease or in a new disease area begin to happen at this point. Price expectations and mode of administration are taken into account, in some cases disease-specific formulations of the same product are developed.

Decision to withdraw/reduce promotional spend

This decision is based upon time to patent expiry, emergent competitor data, and price pressure. Highly validated models exist that predict the impact of promotional spend based on years in market, number of competitors, etc.; these are used to drive any reduction/withdrawal of promotional activity.

Fixed dose combination products (FDC)

Fixed dose combinations have been successfully used to extend the sales life of an innovator compound in a number of cases. These may be FDCs combining two existing agents, or ones combining the agent which is reaching the end of its patent life with an NCE. Companies choose to follow this path because it discourages switching to a cheaper generic, but it is doubtful whether these strategies represent real clinical innovation.

Decision to move prescription-only medicine to pharmacy medicine or pharmacy medicine to general sales list

These decisions are taken in consultation with the regulatory authorities, and may extend the brand heritage of a previously successful prescription-only medicine. Only medicines which have a very well characterized safety profile, for an indication where members of the public frequently request a pharmacy consultation or purchase over the counter, are considered for switching. Examples include Zantac (ranitidine) for the treatment of indigestion, Viagra (sildenafil) for the treatment of erectile dysfunction, and Zocor (simvastatin) for reduction of cardiovascular risk in patients who don't meet the guidelines for NHS-funded treatment of statin therapy.

Ethical marketing of medicines

Overview

In order to inform healthcare professionals about new treatment options available and to enable them to provide the most appropriate treatment for their patients, promotion of medicines is an essential activity. It is also important to allow companies to gain adequate return on the significant R&D investment within the period of patent protection and market exclusivity so that they can continue to invest in new treatments.

However, given the unique nature of advertising medicines, the pharmaceutical industry has an obligation to communicate health information with integrity, accuracy, clarity, and completeness. This ethical obligation goes above and beyond any legal requirements.

Ethical promotion helps to ensure that:
- Healthcare professionals have access to information they need.
- Patients have access to the medicines they need.
- Medicines are prescribed and used in a manner that provides the maximum healthcare benefit to patients.

Therefore, upholding these principles in communications with all stakeholders is very important. How the pharmaceutical industry regulates its communication and interaction with the healthcare professionals is a critical application of this responsibility.

The World Health Organization

The WHO Ethical Criteria on Medicinal Drug Promotion was issued in 1988. The main objective of these ethical criteria was to support and encourage the improvement of healthcare through the rational use of medicinal drugs.

It was accepted that, while the interpretation of what is ethical varies in different parts of the world and in different societies, the issue in all societies is, What is proper behaviour? Ethical criteria for drug promotion should lay the foundation for proper behaviour concerning the promotion of medicinal drugs, 'consistent with the search for truthfulness and righteousness.' The criteria should thus assist in judging if promotional practices related to medicinal drugs are in keeping with acceptable ethical standards.

These criteria constitute general principles for ethical standards which could be adapted by governments to national circumstances. They apply to prescription and non-prescription medicinal drugs ('over-the-counter drugs'). They also apply generally to traditional medicines as appropriate, and to any other product promoted as a medicine.

The criteria do not constitute legal obligations but governments may adopt legislation or other measures based on them as they deem fit. Similarly, other groups may adopt self-regulatory measures based on them. All these bodies should monitor and enforce their standards.

To this end a number of self-regulation instruments have developed to govern the promotion of pharmaceutical products to healthcare professionals—including doctors, pharmacists, and nurses.

The IFPMA Code of Pharmaceutical Marketing Practices was the first international self-regulation mechanism in the pharmaceutical industry, preceding even the WHO's ethical criteria on medicinal drug promotion.

Further reading

WHO Expert Committee on the Use of Essential Drugs. *The Use of Essential Drugs*: second report (WHO Technical Report Series, No. 722, 1985, p. 43).

The World Health Organization ethical criteria for medicinal drug promotion

The World Health Organization

The WHO is the directing and co-ordinating authority for health within the United Nations and is responsible for providing leadership on global health matters, shaping the health research agenda, setting norms and standards, articulating evidence-based policy options, providing technical support to countries, and monitoring and assessing health trends.

Medicinal product promotion

The main objective of the WHO criteria for ethical medicinal drug promotion is to encourage and support the improvement of healthcare through the rational use of medicinal products. The criteria attempt to lay down a common foundation for proper behaviour, consistent with the concepts of righteousness and truthfulness. Therefore, the criteria help to determine correct promotional practices, in keeping with acceptable ethical standards.

The criteria represent general principles for ethical standards and apply to both prescription and non-prescription medicinal products. The criteria may apply to anyone involved in medicinal drug promotion. The criteria define promotion as 'all informational and persuasive activities by manufacturers and distributors, the effect of which is to induce the prescription, supply, purchase and/or use of medicinal drugs.'

The following apply to the promotion of medicinal products:
- Active promotion within a country should take place only with respect to legally available drugs.
- Promotion should be in keeping with national health policies and in compliance with national regulations, including voluntary standards.
- All promotional claims should be:
  - Reliable.
  - Accurate.
  - Truthful.
  - Informative.
  - Balanced.
  - Up-to-date.
  - Capable of substantiation.
  - In good taste.
  - Fully consistent with the approved scientific data sheet.
- Promotional material should not contain misleading or unverifiable statements or important omissions.
- The word 'safe' should only be used if properly qualified.
- Comparison of products should be factual, fair, and capable of substantiation.
- Promotional material should not be designed so as to disguise its true purpose.
- Financial or material benefits should not be offered to or sought by healthcare practitioners to influence the prescription of drugs.
- Scientific and educational activities should not be deliberately used for promotional purposes.

Other considerations include:
- Where acceptable, advertisements to the general public should seek to help people to make rational decisions about their health.
- Medical representatives should have an appropriate educational background and should be adequately trained.
- Free samples of legally available prescription drugs may be provided in modest quantities to prescribers, generally on request.
- The fact symposia and other scientific meetings are sponsored by a pharmaceutical manufacturer or distributor should be clearly stated in advance, at the meeting and in any proceedings.

Further reading

WHO. Available at: ℜ http://apps.who.int/medicinedocs/en/d/Js16520e/16.1.html

Co-marketing and co-promotion

Co-marketing

A co-marketing agreement involves two or more separate companies agreeing to market and sell an identical product, but under two different brand names. This allows for marketing space, and often by companies adopting their own marketing style, increases the share of voice and thus overall market share.

If the molecule has more than one indication, it is possible for the agreement to specify that each company can only market one of the indications, which can reduce the competition for market share by the same molecule.

Co-marketing is sometimes difficult with respect to sales force planning, and often one company's sales force may find a competitor has visited only a few minutes before. Regional agreements and profit sharing agreements can, however, overcome many of these problems.

Co-promotion

A co-promotion agreement is where the marketing authorization holder agrees with another organization to contract further resource to aid promotion. The major difference is that the original marketing authorization holder retains responsibility for many of the activities around the manufacture, marketing, sales, and adverse event reporting for that particular medicine, and the activities of the co-promoter are usually subsidiary to the marketing authorization holder

Division of key responsibilities

Key responsibilities are around the reporting of adverse events. Where co-marketing agreements exist, adverse events may be reported via both companies, and EU medicines law requires adverts or marketing materials to include a telephone number/contact details for this purpose. Periodic safety update reports are usually compiled by one lead company, with input from or access to data from the other partner. With respect to co-promotion agreements the marketing authorization holder is solely responsible for collation and reporting of adverse events.

Where co-promotion exists, complaints around marketing materials are usually made to the marketing authorization holder, although complaints about sales activities or scientific engagement activities may occur to both parties. In co-marketing, the individual companies are responsible for all of their own materials/activities.

Examples of successful co-promotion

A number of examples of successful co-promotion exist, Japanese company Takeda, at the point of their first entry to the UK market formed a number of co-promotion agreements, including with Astra-Zeneca around the promotion of Candesartan. Co-marketing agreements are particularly popular in certain European countries, for example Spain, where sitagliptin is marketed as Teseval by Amirall, a local Spanish pharmaceutical manufacturer, and as Januvia by MSD. This is done by international manufacturers to secure both favourable reimbursement, and additional market share.

Chapter 7.7

In-licensing

Overview

Much has been made of the fall off in productivity of traditional big pharma, and one way to potentially bridge gaps in a therapy area portfolio is via in-licensing. Increasingly where companies have a particular disease area franchise supported by a heritage block buster product or products which are nearing patent expiry, in-licensing is a default option. A number of strategic questions, however, need to be answered prior to even approaching other parties about a potential deal.

Strategic considerations

What are the disease areas which still carry significant unmet need?

Diseases where there has been no significant impact on morbidity or mortality, despite investment in modern pharmaceuticals: For example, significant unmet need exists for heart failure, where in NYHA II functional status or worse, prognosis is worse than that for most tumours.

Is the target disease indication heavily genericized?

Whilst it may not be impossible to launch a new agent for a heavily genericized indication, existing agents will set a price ceiling for reimbursement. As such after taking development costs into account, NPV may not be positive at a low price point.

What in house compounds are available and what stage in development have they reached?

A candid view about the strengths and weaknesses of the in-house portfolio. Timeline of what will be delivered when, and what are the potential gaps. Should any in-licensing agreement be time limited? How should royalties/development costs be structured with respect to timing/probability of success for in-house assets?

What does the competitive landscape look like?

Are there other launches planned by competitors within the timeframe? List the potential differentiators for the potential in-licensed compound vs. the competitors. Without potential differentiation, any opportunity is likely to represent poor value.

Key components of deal structure

- *Steering committee:*
  - Representation from yours and the partner company, voting structure, mechanism for settling disputes.
  - Key responsibility for regulatory filings/clinical development.
  - Joint responsibility for each territory? Split for US/EU/rest of the world? Who is sponsor for each study/each regulatory filing?

- *Marketing authorization:* Who is registered as the holder of marketing authorization? Is this global, regional, or decided on a country-by-country basis?
- *Spend on advertising and promotion:* What is the desired split with respect to spend on A and P? How does this offset/compensate for development costs? Is there a split of promotional spend or a simple royalty agreement?
- *Rules for the end-game:* What are the rules for dissolving the partnership? What are the penalties involved and potential timelines?

Summary

Whilst in-licensing has been seen as the sticking plaster for the fall off in big pharma productivity, there are important considerations with respect to the strategic fit of any new compound and the deal structure itself. It is important to get both right up front, otherwise significant amounts of money may go astray.

The Association of British Pharmaceutical Industries

Overview

The ABPI represents innovative research-based biopharmaceutical companies, both large and small, which supply 90% of all medicines used by the NHS. It is a government recognized body that negotiates the pricing of branded medicines on behalf of the entire industry. It also promotes the UK as a destination of choice for international life sciences investment.

Objectives

The ABPI seeks to represent the views of the research-based pharmaceutical industry in England, Scotland, Wales, and Northern Ireland, as well as at UK, European, and international levels.

The pivotal role that the pharmaceutical industry has played, and continues to play, in improving the health, well-being, and productivity of the UK population is often underestimated. The objective is to ensure that this is better understood.

They maintain close contacts with government, politicians, academia, and the media and have extensive links with health managers, patient advocacy groups, training and education bodies, research councils, and other professional bodies in the healthcare field.

Core imperatives

Work is centred around four core imperatives:
• Value.
• Innovation.
• Trust.
• Access.

The commercial team is focused on value and access, working to ensure that the value of medicines is properly assessed and understood, that physicians are free to prescribe the best medicines for their patients and therefore, that the right patients receive the right medicines at the right time.

The Medical and Innovation department works closely with research teams and organizations across the UK and beyond, seeking to reinforce the importance of R&D.

The Trust imperative aims to develop a new 'contract' between industry and society based on integrity, honesty, knowledge, transparency, and appropriate behaviour.

The Prescription Medicines Code of Practice Authority (PMCPA)

- The PMCPA administers the ABPI Code of Practice at arm's length from the ABPI itself.
- The ABPI Code covers the promotion of medicines for prescribing to health professionals and the provision of information to the public about prescription only medicines.
- The ABPI Code incorporates the principles set out in the international and European codes. In addition it incorporates the principles set out in WHO ethical criteria for medicinal drug promotion.
- The PMCPA liaises regularly with the IFPMA which operates the International Code of Pharmaceutical Marketing Practices and the EFPIA, which operates the European Code of Practice on the Promotion of Medicines to ensure that the UK Code is in line with these codes as far as national law permits.
- Efficient, stringent, and transparent self-regulation via the ABPI Code enables regulatory requirements to be met by self-regulation. The MHRA will act when there is a clear case for protection or if self-regulation fails.
- Self-regulation should be the first means of dealing with complaints. Both the PMCPA and the MHRA deal with complaints whatever their source. However, the MHRA focus is on pre-vetting, dealing with complaints other than inter-company complaints and dealing with complaints that are not covered by the ABPI Code or other self-regulatory authority. The MHRA can refer complaints to the PMCPA.
- A Memorandum of Understanding setting out the relationship has been agreed between the PMCPA, the ABPI, and the MHRA.

Further reading

ABPI. Available at: http://www.abpi.org.uk/Pages/default.aspx
PMCPA. Available at: http://www.pmcpa.org.uk/?q=howwefitwithothers

The Association of British Pharmaceutical Industries Code of Practice

Overview

The ABPI Code of Practice for the pharmaceutical industry sets standards for advertising and promotion of medicines for prescribing to health professionals and appropriate administrative staff in the UK. It includes requirements for the provision of information on POMs to the general public. In addition, it applies to a number of areas that are non-promotional. However, it does not apply to the promotion of over-the-counter medicines to the general public. PMCPA administers the ABPI Code of Practice at arm's length from the ABPI itself.

What the Code covers

The Code covers a number of areas which are outlined in Box 7.9.1.

Box 7.9.1. What the ABPI Code covers

- Journal and direct mail advertising.
- The activities of representatives, including detail aids and other printed material used by representatives.
- The supply of samples.
- The provisions of inducements to prescribe, supply, administer, buy or sell medicines, by the gift, offer or promise of any benefit or bonus, whether in money or in kind.
- The provision of hospitality.
- Promotional meetings.
- The sponsorship of scientific and other meetings, including payment of travelling, and accommodation expenses.
- All other sales promotion, including exhibitions, electronic media, and the Internet.
- The provision of information to the public about prescription only medicines and pharmaceutical companies' relationships with patient organizations.

Reproduced from The Code of Practice for the Pharmaceutical Industry 2012, Clause 1. Please note that the ABPI Code of Practice is regularly reviewed and new editions are published frequently. Before reliance on what is printed within this chapter, readers should check to see whether the wording of the ABPI Code has changed since this book was first published.

The Code aims to ensure that pharmaceutical companies operate in a responsible, ethical, and professional manner. Compliance with the Code is obligatory for ABPI member companies and, in addition, a number of non-member companies have voluntarily agreed to comply with the Code and to accept the jurisdiction of the PMCPA.

The pharmaceutical industry strongly supports the Code with all companies devoting considerable resources to ensure compliance. Any complaint made against a company under the Code is regarded as a serious matter both by the company and by the industry on a whole. All complaints are investigated. The PMCPA deals with the complaints and sanctions are applied when a breach of the Code is ruled.

Making a complaint

Anyone can make a complaint to the PMCPA under the Code. Complaints submitted under the Code are considered in the first instance by the Code of Practice Panel which consists of the members of the Authority, acting with the assistance of independent expert advisers where appropriate.

Once the parties have been advised of the panel's rulings, brief details are put on the ongoing cases section of the website. Both the complainant and the respondent company may appeal to the Code of Practice Appeal Board against rulings made by the Panel. The Code of Practice Appeal Board is chaired by an independent legally qualified chairman and includes independent members from outside the industry.

Further reading

PMCPA Code of Practice. Available at: ℘ http://www.pmcpa.org.uk/?q=whatiscodeofpractice

Pharmaceutical Research and Manufacturers of America

Overview

The Pharmaceutical Manufacturer's Association (PMA), which represents research-based pharmaceutical and biotechnology companies was
founded in 1958. The name was changed to the Pharmaceutical Research
and Manufacturers of America (PhRMA) in 1994.

PhRMA state that its mission is 'to conduct effective advocacy for public
policies that encourage discovery of important new medicines for patients
by biopharmaceutical research companies.'

The Association is governed by a 31-member Board of Directors and an
18-member Executive Committee.

Membership

There are four categories of membership in PhRMA:

- *Members:* organizations significantly engaged in the manufacture
  and marketing of ethical pharmaceutical or biological products
  and significantly engaged in pharmaceutical, biopharmaceutical, or
  biological research and development of new molecular entities or
  new therapies, preventative, or in vivo diagnostics, or new systems of
  therapy, prevention, or diagnosis and who will continue to conduct
  such research and development.
- *Pharmaceutical affiliates:* organizations that would be eligible for
  membership but for the fact that they have contracted with others to
  significantly engage in the manufacture and/or marketing of the ethical
  pharmaceutical or biological products.
- *International affiliates:* organizations not eligible for membership which
  are the subsidiary in the USA of a foreign corporation that is engaged
  in discovery, research, manufacture, and marketing of pharmaceutical
  or biological products.
- *Associate:* organizations not eligible for membership, but who are
  engaged in research and development, in supplying members with
  contract research and development services, Providers to members
  of advertising or communications services to the health professions
  or firms (a) that make and supply members with drug discovery
  software, or (b) that are significantly engaged in providing members
  with consulting services in management, marketing, and information
  management directly related to the manufacture, marketing, or
  research and development of ethical pharmaceutical or biological
  products.

Code of Practice

PhRMA adopts a voluntary Code on relationships with US healthcare professionals. This Code reflects the standards and principles on interactions with healthcare professionals, and addresses interactions with respect to marketed products and related pre-launch activities.

PhRMA member companies' relationships with clinical investigators and other individuals and entities as they relate to the clinical research process are addressed in the PhRMA Principles on Conduct of Clinical Trials and Communication of Clinical Trial Results.

The Code dictates that promotional materials provided to healthcare professionals by or on behalf of a company should:
- Be accurate and not misleading.
- Make claims about a product only when properly substantiated.
- Reflect the balance between risks and benefits.
- Be consistent with all other Food and Drug Administration (FDA) requirements governing such communications.

The PhRMA Code is laid out under the headings shown in Box 7.10.1.

Box 7.10.1 Areas covered by the PhRMA Code
- Informational presentations by pharmaceutical company.
- Representatives and accompanying meals.
- Prohibition on entertainment and recreation.
- Pharmaceutical company support for continuing medical education.
- Pharmaceutical company support for third-party.
- Educational or professional meetings.
- Consultants.
- Speaker programmes and speaker training meetings.
- Healthcare professionals who are members of committees that set formularies or develop clinical practice guidelines.
- Scholarships and educational funds.
- Prohibition of non-educational and practice-related items.
- Educational items.
- Prescriber data.
- Independence and decision making.
- Training and conduct of company representatives.

Chapter 7.11

The International Federation of Pharmaceutical Manufacturers & Associations Code of Practice

Overview

The IFPMA Code of Practice shares core principles with the European code of pharmaceutical marketing practice, and various single country codes of practice. The Code has evolved into a self-regulatory instrument to govern the promotion of pharmaceutical products to healthcare professionals—including doctors, pharmacists, and nurses. It follows several core principles:

- *Basis of interaction:* relationships with healthcare professionals are intended to benefit patients and to enhance the practice of medicine; interactions should be focused on informing healthcare professionals about products, providing scientific and educational information and supporting medical research and education.
- *Independence of healthcare professionals:* healthcare professionals should not be influenced to prescribe, recommend, purchase, supply, or administer a product because of any benefits offered (financial or otherwise).
- *Appropriate use:* promotion should encourage the appropriate use of pharmaceutical products by presenting them objectively and without exaggeration.
- *Local regulations:* all relevant laws, local regulations, and industry codes must be observed.

Transparency of promotion

- All company-sponsored material relating to pharmaceutical products and their uses should clearly indicate by whom it has been sponsored; clinical assessments, post-marketing surveillance, and experience programmes, and post-authorization studies must be conducted with a primarily scientific or educational purpose.
- The IFPMA Code applies to all pharmaceutical products, including prescription, generic and OTC medicines that are promoted to healthcare professionals by member companies worldwide.
- Adherence to and compliance with the Code is a condition of IFPMA membership.
- In the event of a conflict between the IFPMA Code and local laws or regulations, member associations must adopt codes that meet local requirements, but are consistent with and at least as comprehensive as the IFPMA Code.
- For countries where there is no national code, the IFPMA Code supplies one.
- Compliance is monitored and promoted by a Code Compliance Network (CCN), which gathers worldwide experts to discuss the latest developments and issues in the field of ethical promotion of medicines.

Further reading

ACCC Code of Conduct. Available at: ℅ http://www.ifpma.org/fileadmin/content/About%20us/2%20Members/Associations/Code-Austraria/1_AUS-EN-Code-2010[1].pdf

Chapter 7.12

The European Federation of Pharmaceutical Industries and Associations

Overview

The EFPIA is the representative body of the pharmaceutical industry in Europe. Its members are the national industry associations of 30 countries in Europe and over 40 leading pharmaceutical companies. EFPIA states that its primary mission is to promote the technological and economic development of the pharmaceutical industry in Europe and to assist in bringing to market medicinal products which improve human health.

Priorities

EFPIA has focused its priorities around four key areas—the AIMS (Access, Innovation, Mobilization, and Security) programme:

- Access refers to working towards speeding up regulatory approval and reimbursement processes for new medicines—removing government controls on medicines that are not reimbursed and ensure that Health Technology Assessment (HTA) does not become a hurdle to market access.
- Innovation focuses on creating a strong science base in Europe and making Europe an attractive location for the best researchers ensuring a fair reward for innovation and ensuring a high level of protection for intellectual property rights.
- Mobilization is about working with key stakeholders to address the challenges of an ageing population, and deliver modern and sustainable healthcare to fight cost-containment policies to empower patients and citizens to take an active role in managing their health through better access to information from multiple sources to highlight industry's contribution to access to medicines and to promote new incentives for research into diseases affecting the developing world.
- Security refers to the need to strengthen the integrity and transparency of the pharmaceutical supply chain by addressing the safety concerns of parallel trade—raising public awareness on the risk of counterfeits and increasing the traceability of pharmaceutical products.

In order to ensure that relationships between the pharmaceutical industry and patient organizations take place in an ethical and transparent manner, EFPIA has adopted the EFPIA Code of Practice on Relationships between the Pharmaceutical Industry and Patient Organizations.

This Code builds upon the following principles (Box 7.12.1) that EFPIA, together with pan-European patient organizations, last updated in September 2006:

Box 7.12.1 Principles of the EFPIA Code of Practice on relationships between the pharmaceutical industry and patient organisations

- The independence of patient organisations, in terms of their political judgement, policies and activities, shall be assured.
- All partnerships between patient organisations and the pharmaceutical industry shall be based on mutual respect, with the views and decisions of each partner having equal value.
- The pharmaceutical industry shall not request, nor shall patient organisations undertake, the promotion of a particular prescription-only medicine.
- The objectives and scope of any partnership shall be transparent. Financial and non-financial support provided by the pharmaceutical industry shall always be clearly acknowledged.
- The pharmaceutical industry welcomes broad funding of patient organisations from multiple sources.

Reproduced with permission from the European Federation of Pharmaceutical Industries and Associations, 'EFPIA Code of Practice on the relationships between the pharmaceutical industry and patient organisations', 2012. The full text of the Code is available at: ℅ www. efpia.eu.

EFPIA and its members are conscious of the importance of providing accurate, fair, and objective information about medicinal products so that rational decisions can be made as to their use. With this in mind, EFPIA has adopted the EFPIA Code on the Promotion of Prescription-Only Medicines to, and Interactions with, Healthcare Professionals (the 'EFPIA Code'). The EFPIA Code reflects the requirements of council Directive 2001/83/EC relating to medicinal products for human use (the 'Directive'). The EFPIA Code fits into the general framework established by the Directive, which recognizes the role of voluntary control of advertising of medicinal products by self-regulatory bodies and recourse to such bodies when complaints arise. The EFPIA Code seeks to ensure that pharmaceutical companies conduct promotion and interaction in a truthful manner, avoiding deceptive practices and potential conflicts of interest with healthcare professionals, and in compliance with applicable laws and regulations.

Further reading

EFPIA. EFPIA vision. Available at: ℅ http://www.efpia.org/Content/Default.asp?PageID=319

Medicines Australia

Overview

Medicines Australia represents the pharmaceutical industry in Australia. Its member companies supply 86% of the medicines that are available to Australian patients through the Pharmaceutical Benefits Scheme, as well as providing a range of other medicines and vaccines to the Australian community.

Medicines Australia represents the industry by:
- Engaging with government and government departments, the Australian medicines industry, consumer groups, and health professionals to develop health and industry policy.
- Building and maintaining relationships with government for fair reimbursement of medicines (through the Pharmaceuticals Benefits Scheme) to ensure the continuation of a viable medicines industry.
- Administering the Medicines Australia Code of Conduct, which sets the standard for the ethical marketing and promotion of prescription medicines.
- Working with other health professional and consumer organizations on issues of mutual concern.
- Providing specialist advice to member companies.
- Educating the community about industry activities.

The Code of Conduct

Adherence to the Code of Conduct is a requirement of membership of Medicines Australia. The Code of Conduct sets the standards for the ethical marketing and promotion of prescription pharmaceutical products in Australia. It complements the legislation requirements of the Therapeutic Goods Regulations and the Therapeutic Goods Act.

Code provisions include standards for appropriate advertising, the behaviour of medical representatives, and relationships with healthcare professionals. Medicines Australia's Code of Conduct, which was established in 1960, has been revised on a regular basis to ensure that the Code continues to reflect current community and professional standards and current government legislation. It is now in its 16th edition.

Areas covered by the Code of Conduct include:
- *Nature and availability of information and claims:* false and misleading claims, level of substantiating data.
- Types of product information.
  - *Promotional material:* advertisements, brand name reminders, competitions, gifts, and offers.
  - *Company representatives:* medical representatives.
- Product starter packs.
- *Involvement in educational symposia, congresses, and satellite meetings:* trade displays.
- Sponsorship.
- Research.
- Relationship with the general public.
- *Relationship with healthcare professionals:* travel, hospitality, remuneration, entertainment, consultants, and advisory boards.
- Educational events.
- *Administration of the code:* complaints process, committee membership.
- Sanctions.
- Appeals.
- Monitoring.
- Compliance procedures.
- Reporting.

The Code of Conduct Committee, with medical, legal, and consumer representatives, has the power to order withdrawal of advertising, require letters of clarification, and impose company fines for breaches of the Code.

Further reading

Medicines Australia. Issues/Information. Available at: ℅ http://medicinesaustralia.com.au/issues-information

Chapter 7.14

National Institute for Health and Clinical Excellence

Overview

The NICE is a Special Health Authority—an arm's length body funded by the Department of Health. It was set up in 1999 to reduce variation in the availability and quality of NHS treatments and care.

Their evidence-based guidance, evidence-based guidelines, and other products help resolve uncertainty about which medicines, treatments, procedures, and devices represent the best quality care and which offer the best value for money for the NHS.

Structure

NICE is structured around 4 directorates and 3 centres:
- *Clinical and public health directorate:* oversees:
  - Research and development.
  - Information service.
  - Patient and Public Involvement Programme (PPIP).
- Communications directorate.
- Implementation directorate.
- *Business, planning, and resources directorate:*
  - Centre for public health excellence.
  - Develops guidance on the promotion of good health and the prevention of ill health.
- *Centre for health technology evaluation:* develops guidance on the use of new and existing medicines, treatments, and procedures within the NHS.
- *Centre for clinical practice:* develops clinical guidelines on the appropriate treatment and care of people with specific diseases or conditions for people working in the NHS.

Health technology appraisal

The appraisal of a health technology is divided into three distinct phases.
- *Scoping:* during the scoping process, the Institute determines the appropriateness of the remit and the specific questions that are to be addressed for each technology appraisal. Consultees and commentators are consulted during the scoping process. The Institute revises the scope in response to comments received and develops a final scope that describes the boundaries of the appraisal and the issues that will be investigated.
- *Assessment:* the assessment process is a systematic evaluation of the relevant evidence available on a technology. Assessment normally has two mutually dependent components: a systematic review of the evidence and an economic evaluation. Strengths, weaknesses, and gaps in the evidence are identified and evaluated. The assessment process always includes a review of the evidence by an independent assessment group. They may recommend that the Institute requests

additional analysis from the manufacturer or sponsor, and may undertake sensitivity analysis.
- *Appraisal:* the appraisal process is a consideration of the reports and analyses produced in the assessment phase. The Appraisal Committee considers the evidence available and then formulates an appraisal decision, applying judgements on the importance of a range of factors that may differ from appraisal to appraisal.

Fundamental principles

- The Institute takes into account the clinical and cost effectiveness of a technology, when issuing guidance to the NHS.
- In general, technologies can be considered clinically effective if they confer an overall health benefit.
- Technologies can be considered to be cost effective if their health benefits are greater than the opportunity costs measured in terms of the health benefits associated with programmes that may be displaced to fund the new technology.
- The Institute is committed to promoting equality, eliminating unlawful discrimination, and actively considering the implications of its guidance for human rights.

Implementation of NICE guidance

The implementation of NICE guidance is a legal requirement. The Secretary of State for Health has directed that the NHS provides funding and resources for technologies that have been recommended through the NICE technology appraisals programme, normally within 3 months from the date that the guidance is published.

Further reading

NICE. Available at: ℘ http://www.nice.org.uk/

The Scottish Intercollegiate Guidelines Network

Overview

The Scottish Intercollegiate Guidelines Network (SIGN) develops evidence-based clinical practice guidelines for the NHS in Scotland. SIGN guidelines are derived from a systematic review of the scientific literature and are designed as a vehicle for accelerating the translation of new knowledge into action. The objective is to improve the quality of healthcare for patients in Scotland by reducing variation in practice and outcome, through the development and dissemination of national clinical guidelines containing recommendations for effective practice based on current evidence.

Since 1 January 2005 SIGN has been part of NHS Quality Improvement Scotland. The membership of SIGN includes:
- All the medical specialties.
- Nursing.
- Pharmacy.
- Dentistry.
- Professions allied to medicine.
- Patients.
- Health service managers.
- Social services.
- Researchers.

Guideline development process

Any group or individual can propose a topic for a SIGN guideline. For a topic to be suitable for the development of a SIGN guideline there must be evidence of variation in practice which affects patient outcomes and a strong research base providing evidence of effective practice. In addition, the potential benefit to patients must be sufficient to justify the resources invested in the development and implementation of a SIGN guideline.

SIGN guidelines are developed by multidisciplinary working groups with representation from across Scotland. The guideline development groups are selected in consultation with the member organizations of SIGN Council. Each guideline is based on a systematic review and critical appraisal of the current scientific literature. This means that the evidence base for the guideline is identified, selected, and evaluated according to a defined methodology. In this way, potential sources of bias in the guideline are minimized and the likely validity of the recommendations is maximized. The guideline recommendations are graded according to the strength of the supporting evidence. This provides groups of practitioners working in NHS Scotland with information to help select and prioritize recommendations for local implementation, depending on local needs, priorities, and resources.

All SIGN guidelines are also independently reviewed by specialist referees prior to publication. Three years after publication (or sooner if required) the guideline is formally considered for review and is updated where necessary to take account of newly published evidence.

Dissemination and implementation

SIGN guidelines are distributed within the NHS in Scotland via a network of Guideline Distribution Co-ordinators in each NHS Board. Implementation is the responsibility of each individual NHS Board.

SIGN is also working collaboratively with the NHS QIS Implementation and Improvement Support Directorate to support putting evidence into practice and to drive the improvement of health services.

Further reading

SIGN. Available at: ℘ http://www.sign.ac.uk/about/index.html

The Institute for Quality and Efficiency in Health Care

Overview

The Institute for Quality and Efficiency in Health Care (IQWiG) is an independent scientific institute that investigates the benefits and harms of medical interventions for patients in Germany. The Institute produces independent, evidence-based reports on:

- Drugs.
- Non-drug interventions (e.g. surgical procedures).
- Diagnostic tests and screening tests.
- Clinical practice guidelines (CPGs) and disease management programmes (DMPs).

In addition IQWiG provides health information for the general public. The sole contracting agencies are the Federal Joint Committee (GBA) and the Federal Ministry of Health (BMG). IQWiG can also select topics on its own initiative (general commission).

Structure

IQWiG is composed of eight departments. These include:

- Drug assessment.
- Non-drug interventions.
- Quality of healthcare.
- Medical biometry.
- Health economics.
- Health information.
- Administration.
- Communication.

Work principles

IQWiG works under the following guiding principles:

- *Independence:* the Institute carries out its scientific work in an independent manner. The contents of the reports cannot be influenced by those in industry, the statutory health insurance funds or politics.
- *Objective and evidence-based:* IQWiG reports are not based on personal opinions or convictions, but on proof.
- *Patient-oriented:* when assessing benefit, IQWiG applies criteria that are important to patients.
- *Transparent:*
  - IQWiG not only publishes the final reports on its projects, but also the intermediate stages, such as the draft of the report plan, and the preliminary results (preliminary report).
  - Scientists, industry, professional societies, doctors, and patients have the opportunity to submit comments on IQWiG's work at different stages in the project.
- *Scientific:* in its role as scientific institute, IQWiG also maintains a regular exchange with other research institutes and networks.

Product-specific procedures

The product range of the Institute includes four main products:
- Detailed reports (especially benefit and cost–benefit assessments).
- Rapid reports.
- Health information (easily understandable information for consumers and patients).
- Working papers (on relevant healthcare developments and on the Institute's methodological work).

Detailed reports procedure

After commissioning by the GBA or BMG, the research question is developed in consultation with the contracting agency's responsible committees, involving external professional expertise.
- A report plan containing the precise scientific research question is produced. This preliminary report plan is then forwarded to the contracting agency and is then published on the Institute's website (usually 5 working days later), in order to provide the opportunity to submit comments.
- For a period of at least 4 weeks, the public and other stakeholders are given the opportunity to submit written comments. The opportunity is also provided to submit any type of document of appropriate quality (especially unpublished data), which is suited to answer the research question of the report.
- After the analysis of the comments, the revised report plan is published. This report plan is the basis for the preparation of the preliminary report.
- The results of the literature search and the scientific assessment are presented in the preliminary report. The preliminary report includes the preliminary recommendation to the Federal Joint Committee. It is produced under the responsibility of the IQWiG project group, usually with the involvement of external experts.
- The preliminary report is published on the Institute's website (usually 5 working days after delivery to the contracting agency) in order to provide the public the opportunity to submit comments (hearing procedure) for a period of at least 4 weeks.
- The final report, which is based upon the preliminary report and contains the assessment of the scientific findings (considering the results of the hearing), represents the concluding product of the work on the commission.

Further reading

IQWiG. Available at: ℛ https://www.iqwig.de/index.2.en.html

Health economics

Overview

Health economics is a branch of economics concerned with issues related to scarcity in the allocation of health and healthcare. Health economics studies how healthcare and health-related services, their costs and benefits, and health itself are distributed among individuals and groups in society. Health economics is concerned with the formal analysis of direct and indirect costs and benefits that are a consequence of a healthcare intervention, programme, or strategy. Health economics has some distinct differences from other branches of economics. These include:

• Significant government intervention.
• Uncertainty that is intrinsic to health.
• *Asymmetry of information:* the asymmetry of information makes the relationship between patients and doctors rather different from the usual relationship between buyers and sellers. We rely upon our doctor to act in our best interests, to act as our agent. However, they must also act in their own interests as the seller of healthcare.
• *Externalities:* knowing that someone is in pain simply because they cannot afford medical treatment makes many people upset. In other words, the poor sick person's pain and lack of treatment causes disutility for other people in society. This helps to explain also why some people are prepared to pay higher taxes to fund healthcare for all. Again, a market demand curve reflecting each individual's wish to buy care for themselves is unable to express this willingness to pay for external benefits.

Economic evaluation of a healthcare intervention is the comparison of two or more alternative courses of action in terms of both their costs and consequences. Economists usually distinguish several types of economic evaluation, differing in how consequences are measured:

• Cost–minimization analysis.
• Cost–benefit analysis.
• Cost–effectiveness analysis.
• Cost–utility analysis.

Cost–minimization analysis

This is often considered to be the easiest evaluation to apply as it should only be utilized in situations where the benefits of alternative treatments have been proven to be identical. Therefore, the focus can be entirely on cost. However, the data supporting the assumption of equivalent clinical benefit must be robust and unambiguous before such a complete focus on costs can be justified. For a cost–minimization analysis to be a valid and reliable source of evidence to decision-makers requires the availability of high-quality clinical evidence that proves the equivalence of two treatments and, therefore, indicates the appropriateness of this method of economic evaluation.

Cost–benefit analysis

Cost–benefit analysis (CBA) involves comparing the total expected costs of each intervention against the total expected benefits, to see whether the benefits outweigh the costs, and by how much. Therefore, in CBA, benefits and costs are expressed in money terms. While the costs of an intervention are usually financial and rather easy to quantify, benefits must also be expressed in monetary terms, and this is often very difficult. Indeed, it may be inadequate as using this model does not allow us to accurately put a value on a human life due to the inherent bias that exists in this.

Cost-effectiveness analysis

Cost-effectiveness analysis has been defined by NICE as an economic study design in which consequences of different interventions are measured using a single outcome, usually in 'natural' units (for example, quality-adjusted life years (QALY) gained, deaths avoided). Alternative interventions are then compared in terms of cost per unit of effectiveness.

The assessment of cost-effectiveness is an essential component in determining whether a therapy is approved for reimbursement and for formulary inclusion. HTA agencies, such as NICE, place considerable weight on the relative cost-effectiveness of therapies in making their judgements. NICE requires the use of cost–utility analysis, in which the outcome measure is expressed as a QALY, and which enables comparisons to be made across therapeutic areas—using the QALY as the 'common currency'.

Cost–utility analysis

CUA can be considered a special case of cost-effectiveness analysis, and the two terms are often used interchangeably. In health economics the purpose of CUA is to estimate the ratio between the cost of a health-related intervention and the benefit it produces in terms of the number of years lived in full health by the beneficiaries. Cost is measured in monetary units. Benefit needs to be expressed in a way that allows health states that are considered less preferable to full health to be given quantitative values. In HTAs it is usually expressed in QALYs. CUA allows comparison across different health programmes and policies by using a common unit of measure. However, in CUA societal benefits and costs are often not taken into account. Furthermore, some economists believe that measuring QALYs is more difficult than measuring the monetary value of life through health improvements.

Further reading

National Institute for Health and Clinical Excellence. Guide to the methods of technology appraisal. ℘ www.nice.org.uk/media/B52/A7/TAMethodsGuideUpdatedJune2008.pdf.

Quality-adjusted life years

Overview

The outcomes from treatments and other health-influencing activities have two basic components—the quantity and the quality of life. The QALY captures both the quality and quantity elements of a healthcare outcome in a single arithmetic measure.

The quantity of life, expressed in terms of survival or life expectancy, is widely accepted and has few problems of comparison—people are either alive or not. Quality of life (QOL), on the other hand, embraces a whole range of different facets of people's lives, not just their health status.

Approaches to measure QALYs

A number of approaches can be used to generate these quality of life valuations that are often referred to as health utilities; for example, the use of rating scales. Health utilities are produced with valuations attached to each health state on a continuum between 0 and 1, where 0 is equivalent to being dead and 1 represents the best possible health. Although one treatment might help someone live longer, it might also have serious side effects. (For example, it might make them feel sick, put them at risk of other illnesses, or leave them permanently disabled). Another treatment might not help someone to live as long, but it may improve their quality of life while they are alive (for example, by reducing their pain or disability) (see Box 7.18.1).

> **Box 7.18.1 Example**
> - Treatment A: 3 years in health state 0.5 = 1.5 QALYs
> - Treatment B: 5 years in health state 0.2 = 1.0 QALYs
> - Additional QALYs by treatment A = 0.5 QALYs

Therefore, a treatment that generates 3 additional years in a health state valued at 0.5 will generate 0.5 more QALY than an intervention that generates 5 additional years in a health state valued at 0.2.

When data relating to both health-related quality of life and survival are available, it is then possible to chart the impact of a healthcare intervention on an individual patient. It is also possible to calculate the cost of each additional QALY should we know the cost of the intervention. Therefore, QALYs offer the possibility of carrying out effective cost benefit analysis and thus providing the information we need to make efficient decisions.

Problems with QALYs

While QALYs provide a solution to solve the problem of measuring healthcare outcomes, they suffer from a number of serious problems:

- QALYs are likely to undervalue healthcare because they fail to capture the wider benefits (externalities) that may be gained, for example, by a patient's family and friends.
- Who is to make the subjective choices which determine the QALY? Data has shown that the value of a QALY can change radically according to who is making the choices.
- Other problems include the fact that responses given are to hypothetical situations and may not accurately reflect people's real decisions.
- Valuations are influenced by the length of the illness and the way in which the questions are asked.
- Preventive measures, where the impact on health outcomes may not occur for many years, may be difficult to quantify using QALYs.
- Chronic diseases, where quality of life is a major issue and survival less of an issue, are difficult to accommodate in the QALY.

Nevertheless, the use of QALYs in resource allocation decisions assists commissioners in prioritizing their expenditure against an incessant flow of new technologies and therapies that all claim to enhance the health status of particular patient groups.

Pharmacoepidemiology

Overview

Pharmacoepidemiology (PE) can be defined as the study of the use and effects of drugs in populations. It applies the methods of epidemiology to the area of clinical pharmacology.

Premarketing studies are limited by size, meaning larger studies are required to detect less common adverse effects. The importance of PE lies in the fact that the drug approval process cannot detect adverse events that are relatively uncommon, delayed, specific to high risk populations, etc.

PE studies can, therefore, contribute information about drug safety, which will not be captured by the pre-licence clinical development programme.

Drivers for pharmacoepidemiology studies

The decision to carry out a PE study involves weighing the costs and risks of a therapy against its potential benefits.

However, the decision has 4 main drivers (see Box 7.19.1).

> **Box 7.19.1 Drivers for pharmacoepidemiology studies**
> - Regulatory.
> - Clinical.
> - Marketing.
> - Legal.

Regulatory drivers

A PE study may be required as a condition of granting marketing authorization. Indeed, the manufacturer may offer to carry out a study in anticipation of being granted earlier marketing authorization. A PE study may also be requested in response to reported adverse events. A manufacturer may also carry out a PE study in order to demonstrate safety and aid approval in other regions.

Clinical drivers

The primary clinical driver for a PE study is hypothesis testing. There may be hypothetical problems anticipated based on the chemical structure of the specific class of the medicine. Similarly there may be some undetermined signals during the development process that may require a larger study to test this. This also serves to better quantify the frequency of adverse events. Hypothesis-generating studies may also be required such as in the case of new chemical entities.

Legal drivers

All drugs cause adverse effects. The approval is based on a balance of the benefits and risks. PE studies can therefore be used to protect from future litigation.

Marketing drivers

While PE studies are done for regulatory or clinical reasons, there are clear benefits from a marketing perspective. Prescribers will be more confident in using a medicine with the knowledge of experience and safety data obtained from PE studies. It can also provide some differentiation from competitor products. PE studies can provide answers regarding the safety of a medicine which arise in the marketplace and will therefore, protect the product.

Benefit of pharmacoepidemiology

There are a number of benefits of PE which are summarized in Box 7.19.2.

Box 7.19.2 Benefits of PE

- Fulfils regulatory requirements.
- Better quantification of:
  - Adverse events.
  - Beneficial effects.
  - Effects in unstudied populations (elderly, pregnancy, children, etc.).
  - Interactions with other medicines.
- Better understanding of:
  - Effect of overdose.
  - Patterns of utilization.
  - New adverse events.
  - Economic impact.
  - Reassurance regarding safety.

Chapter 7.20

Branded generics

Overview

Historical attitudes to divestment of branded pharmaceuticals, where all resource is withdrawn post patent expiry have been replaced by continued investment, albeit at a lower level. This has largely been driven by a massive expansion in medical care in the BRIC countries (Brazil, Russia, China, and India), where an ever-expanding middle class wants access to medicines that are dependable with respect to quality.

Where a medicine carries significant heritage, and has extensive clinical trial outcome data, it makes business sense to launch off patent medicines as branded generics, maintaining the name used to promote the medicine during its patent life, and pricing the medicine just above the price charged for locally produced medicines.

As wealth continues to increase in the BRIC countries, so does the burden of non-communicable disease, particularly Type 2 diabetes and cardiovascular disease, the two diseases most associated with large outcome studies.

What makes an ideal branded generic?

- Potentially high area of unmet clinical need, e.g. prevention of cardiovascular disease, blood glucose lowering, hypertension.
- Chemical entity has proven outcome benefit, e.g. simvastatin in cardiovascular outcomes, metformin in blood glucose lowering, ramipril in cardiovascular outcomes.
- Low incidence of drug–drug interactions/favourable toxicity profile.

Combination therapies

Potential added value lies in combining cardiovascular and diabetes medications. Many patients with Type 2 diabetes may be taking 2 oral hypoglycaemic agents, 3 anti-hypertensives, a statin, and one or two anti-platelet agents.

Studies of combination therapies suggest that they may be associated with a compliance benefit of up to 30%, and consequently one would assume greater efficacy.

Routes to market

In some countries a European MA is acceptable. This brings with it the possibility of a substitution application. For a substitution application only demonstration of bioequivalence is necessary, meaning that a relatively small data package is needed to gain registration.

In other countries local data is required; examples of countries where local data is preferred include Korea, Mexico, and Russia, meaning that in these states a study to measure clinical effect is usually undertaken.

Data exclusivity

Increased burden of non-communicable disease also brings with it the possibility of pharmaceutical companies who were not responsible for the innovator product actually registering generic stand-alone or combination products.

One hurdle here, however, is data exclusivity, which may persist post-patent expiry. In practice, this may drive increased need for clinical data with the new generic, and be merely a financial and time barrier to entry, not an insurmountable problem.

Intellectual property

Overview

Intellectual property law is a key consideration with respect to pharmaceutical development. The TRIPS (trade-related aspects of intellectual property rights) agreement now forms the basis for intellectual property law internationally. It is designed to provide incentives for future inventions, whilst maximizing appropriate action to existing ones where possible.

There is flexibility within the agreements for pharmaceutical patents which allow for national emergencies, anti-competitive practices, and failure of the patent holder to supply the product in a particular market.

WTO (World Trade Organization) members are obliged to provide patent protection for any invention, and this should be for a period of 20yrs from the date the patent application was filed.

Patents can be refused for reasons of public health; examples include where commercial exploitation needs to be prevented for reasons of human, animal, or plant health, the patent covers a method of diagnosis, therapy or surgery, which should not be patentable, or a plant or chemical, which should not be patented because it would significantly limit the development of other therapies.

To qualify for a patent, an invention has to be new ('novelty'), it must be an 'inventive step' (i.e. it must not be obvious), and it must have 'industrial applicability' (it must be useful).

Granting of a patent is different to the conditions of registration of a pharmaceutical.

Compulsory licensing

Compulsory licensing is when a government allows someone else to produce the patented product or process without the consent of the patent owner.

The agreement allows compulsory licensing as part of the agreement's overall attempt to strike a balance between promoting access to existing drugs and promoting research and development into new drugs.

Compulsory licensing and government use of a patent without the authorization of its owner can only be done under a number of conditions aimed at protecting the legitimate interests of the patent holder.

For example, normally the person or company applying for a licence must have first attempted, unsuccessfully, to obtain a voluntary licence from the right holder on reasonable commercial terms. If a compulsory licence is issued, adequate remuneration must still be paid to the patent holder.

In cases of national emergency there is no need to have attempted to obtain a voluntary licence first.

Least developed countries

Least developed countries have exemption from the TRIPS agreement, which has recently been extended to 2016 for pharmaceuticals under the Doha agreement for TRIPS and public health. Countries become within scope of the TRIPS agreement once they cease to become least developed.

Further reading

WTO. Developing countries' transition period. Available at: http://www.wto.org/english/tratop_e/trips_e/factsheet_pharm04_e.htm

Product liability and compensation

Overview

With respect to UK law, the consumer protection act from 1987 covers both pharmaceutical products and medical devices.

Such a product will be found to be defective if when supplied, it did not meet the legitimate expectations of those using it, taking into consideration the purpose of the product and any instructions or warnings issued with it. Similar legal frameworks exist for claims in the USA and across most of the countries in Europe. The producer, importer, or supplier of a product will be liable for a defective product on the basis of strict liability where it can be shown that the product was defective and that the defect caused injury. In these circumstances, there is no requirement to prove fault or negligence; however, the producer will escape a claim if they can show that at the time when the product was supplied, the defect was not discoverable within the state of knowledge at that time.

As such, data that becomes apparent after marketing authorization that significantly impacts on benefit risk of the product, and may exclude some patients from appropriate use cannot allow retrospective claims.

If, however, the pharmaceutical company was aware of data that negatively affected the profile of the product and did not make appropriate label changes in conjunction with the regulatory authorities, then a claim for compensation is possible.

Compensation is based around demonstrating any potential loss to the patient. For example, if data from a trial of drug X indicates a significant difference in stroke between it and standard therapy, in favour of standard therapy, a claim against the manufacturer of drug X may be permitted.

Many legal cases centre on opinion, which has been given by employees about early study data on compounds, and whether that opinion constitutes a possible admission of liability.

Opinion written in an email is open to substantial misinterpretation. As such, most organizations now employ 'Write right' courses, whereby employees are taught to write only factual emails and not to include opinion or interpretation if possible.

Further reading

Consumer Protection Act 1987. Available at: ℗ http://www.legislation.gov.uk/ukpga/1987/43

Section 8

Therapeutics

Chapter 8.1

Medicines for children

Paediatric population

Paediatric patients have the same right to well investigated therapies as adults. Paediatric patients should be given medicines that have been appropriately evaluated for their use, and medicines should be prescribed within the terms of a marketing authorization. In Europe, the Paediatric Regulations (Regulation (EC) 1901/2006 and No. 1902/2006) introduced a framework for providing incentives and obligations to companies to conduct research into the use of medicines in the paediatric population. The introduction of the paediatric investigation plan in the legal framework aims at ensuring that the development of medicinal products that are potentially to be used for the paediatric population becomes an integral part of the development of medicinal products.

Special considerations regarding paediatric subjects in clinical studies

When a medicinal product is to be used in the paediatric population for the same indication as approved in adults, some extrapolation from adult efficacy data to the paediatric population may be appropriate. The potential benefit of administering a medicine in the paediatric population should be considered in relation to the risks involved (ICH Topic E11). During the first trimester drugs may produce congenital malformations (greatest risk 3rd–11th week). In the second and third trimester, drugs may affect growth and functional development. The potential for harm from breast-feeding may be inferred from the pharmacokinetic and pharmacodynamic properties of the drug.

The following points should be considered in the paediatric population:

- Paediatric subjects are legally unable to provide informed consent, parents/legal guardians assume responsibility for their participation in clinical studies.
- Children should be involved in decisions about taking medicines.
- Unattractive formulations may contribute to poor compliance and an unpleasant taste may be masked by flavouring.
- Sugar-free medicines should be provided wherever possible.
- Children under 5 may find a liquid formulation more acceptable to tablets.
- The volume of blood withdrawn should be minimized; consider the use of indwelling catheters for repeat sampling.
- For ethical reasons, paediatric pharmacokinetic studies are often performed in patients who may potentially benefit from the treatment.
- The degree of maturation of drug eliminating organs should be considered.
- Discomfort and distress should be minimized.
- Studies should be designed and conducted by investigators experienced in the treatment of paediatric patients.
- Protocols and investigations should be designed specifically for the paediatric population.

Table 8.1.1 Age classification and specific age related issues in clinical development

Age group	Characteristics
Preterm newborn infants	Special challenges because of the unique pathophysiology. Not a homogeneous group of patients. Rapid developmental changes in absorption, distribution, metabolism, and excretion
Term newborn infants (0–27 days)	Volume of distribution may differ from older paediatric patients because of different body water and fat content, and body-surface-area-to-weight ratio. The blood–brain barrier is still not fully mature and medicinal products may gain access to the CNS with resultant toxicity
Infants and toddlers (28 days–23 months)	Characterized by a period of rapid CNS maturation, immune system development, and total body growth. Oral absorption becomes more reliable. Hepatic and renal clearance pathways continue to mature rapidly. By 1–2 years of age, clearance of many drugs may exceed adult values. High inter-individual variability in maturation
Children (2–11yrs)	Hepatic and renal pathways are mature, with clearance often exceeding adult values. Onset of puberty varies markedly between individual children
Adolescents (12–17yrs)	Non-compliance is a special problem. Monitoring the onset of puberty may be important. Consider pregnancy testing, review of sexual activity/contraceptive use as appropriate

- Practical considerations include the physical setting, play equipment, and food appropriate for age.
- It may be necessary to develop, validate, and employ different endpoints for specific age groups.
- Response to a medicinal product may vary because of the developmental stage of the patient.
- Children may be poor at expressing the symptoms of an adverse event, and parental opinion should also be sought.
- Long-term studies or surveillance data may be needed to determine possible effects on skeletal, behavioural, cognitive, sexual, and immune maturation and development.

Further reading

BNF. British National Formulary. Available at: ℘ http://bnf.org/bnf/index.htm

CHMP. Guideline on the role of pharmacokinetics in the development of medicinal products in the paediatric population. Available at: ℘ http://www.ema.europa.eu/docs/en_GB/document_library/Scientific_guideline/2009/09/WC500023066.pdf

ICH. Clinical investigation of medicinal products in the pediatric population—E11. Available at: ℘ http://www.ich.org/fileadmin/Public_Web_Site/ICH_Products/Guidelines/Efficacy/E11/Step4/E11_Guideline.pdf

Medicines in pregnancy

Overview

The physiological changes of pregnancy have the potential to alter the PK and/or PD of drugs. Some of these changes include:
- Changes in total body weight and body fat composition.
- Delayed gastric emptying and prolonged GI transit time.
- Increase in extra cellular fluid and total body water.
- Increased cardiac output, increased stroke volume, and elevated maternal heart rate.
- Decreased albumin concentration with reduced protein binding.
- Increased blood flow to the various organs (e.g. kidneys, uterus).
- Increased glomerular filtration rate.
- Changed hepatic enzyme activity, including phase I CYP450 metabolic pathways (e.g. increased CYP2D6 activity), xanthine oxidase, and phase II metabolic pathways (e.g. N-acetyltransferase).

These will have an effect on how certain drugs are absorbed, metabolized, and excreted.

Drug absorption

High circulating levels of progesterone slow the gastric emptying, as well as gut motility, thus increasing the intestinal transit time. One might expect slower drug absorption during pregnancy for this reason. Administration of iron and antacids may also interfere with the absorption of certain drugs. Drugs compliance may be poor because of nausea and fear of possible adverse effects.

Drug distribution

Pregnancy is accompanied by an increase in total body water by up to 8L and a 30% increase in plasma volume, with consequent decrease in plasma albumin due to haemodilution. Drugs, which have low lipid solubility and are also highly plasma protein bound, have a low apparent volume of distribution (Vd). The Vd of such drugs increases markedly during pregnancy. The protein bound fraction of the drug in the plasma, although the fraction of unbound drug increases, a greater pharmacodynamic effect is prevented by more rapid elimination of drug by metabolism and excretion. The therapeutic range for drugs whose use is monitored by measurement of total plasma concentration must be adjusted downwards to make allowance for the mentioned changes during pregnancy.

Drug metabolism

Hepatic drug metabolizing enzymes are induced during pregnancy, probably by high concentration of circulating progesterone. This can lead to more rapid metabolic degradation, especially of high lipid soluble drugs. The contribution of placenta and fetal liver to the clearance of drugs from the maternal body is thought to be small.

Drug excretion

During pregnancy, the renal plasma flow increases by 100% and the glomerular filtration rate by 70%. Add to this the increase in the unbound fraction of the drug in the plasma. Hence, drugs that depend on their elimination mainly on the kidney are eliminated more rapidly than in the non-pregnant state. Examples of such drugs are ampicillin, gentamycin, cephalexin, and digoxin.

Transplacental transfer

Drugs diffuse across the placenta. Whether and how quickly a drug crosses the placenta depends on the drug's molecular weight, extent of its binding to another substance (e.g. carrier protein), area available for exchange across the villi, and the amount of drug metabolized by the placenta. Most drugs with a molecular weight <500 Daltons readily cross the placenta and enter fetal circulation. Substances with a high molecular weight (e.g. protein-bound drugs) usually do not cross the placenta. The exception is immune globulin G, which is occasionally used to treat disorders such as fetal alloimmune thrombocytopenia. Generally, equilibration between maternal blood and fetal tissues takes at least 40 minutes.

Effect on fetus

A drug's effect on the fetus is determined largely by fetal age at exposure, drug potency, and drug dosage. See Table 8.2.1 for some known or suspected teratogens. Fetal age affects the type of drug effect:

- *Before the 20th day after fertilization:* drugs given at this time may have an all-or-nothing effect, killing the embryo or not affecting it at all. Teratogenesis is not likely during this stage.
- *During organogenesis (between 20 and 56 days after fertilization):* teratogenesis is most likely at this stage. Drugs reaching the embryo at this stage may result in abortion, a sublethal gross anatomic defect (true teratogenic effect), or covert embryopathy (a permanent subtle metabolic or functional defect that may manifest later in life), or the drugs may have no measurable effect.
- *After organogensis (in the 2nd and 3rd trimesters):* teratogenesis is unlikely, but drugs may alter growth and function of normally-formed fetal organs and tissues.

Table 8.2.1 Some known or suspected teratogens

ACE inhibitors	Methimazole
Alcohol	Methotrexate
Aminopterin	Norprogesterones
Androgens	Penicillamine
Carbamazepine	Phenytoin
Coumarins	Radioactive iodine
Danazol	Streptomycin
Diethylstilbestrol	Tetracycline
Etretinate	Thalidomide
Isotretinoin	Trimethadione
Lithium	Valproate

Medicines in the elderly

Overview

Providing safe, effective drug therapy for the elderly is challenging for many reasons:

- They use more drugs, increasing risk of adverse effects and making adherence difficult.
- They are more likely to have chronic disorders that affect drug response.
- Their physiological reserves are reduced.
- Ageing alters pharmacodynamics and pharmacokinetics.

Pharmacokinetic changes with age

With ageing, the absorption, distribution, metabolism, and excretion of many drugs changes, requiring that doses of some drugs be adjusted. See Table 8.3.1 for a summary.

Absorption

Despite an age-related decrease in small bowel surface area, slowed gastric emptying, and an increase in gastric pH, changes in drug absorption tend to be clinically inconsequential for most drugs.

Distribution

In the elderly, there is increased body fat and reduced body water. Increased fat increases the volume of distribution for highly lipophilic drugs and may increase their elimination half-lives, e.g. diazepam. Serum albumin decreases and α1-acid glycoprotein increases with age, but the clinical effect of these changes on serum drug binding is unclear.

Hepatic metabolism

Hepatic metabolism through the cytochrome P-450 enzyme system generally decreases with age. This results in decreased clearance, typically by 30–40%. However, as the rate of drug metabolism varies greatly from person to person, individual titration is required.

Table 8.3.1 Summary of pharmacokinetic changes with age

Decreased	Increased
small-bowel surface area	increase in gastric pH
gastric emptying	increased body fat
body water	increased serum albumin
cytochrome P-450 metabolism	
creatinine clearance	
muscle mass	
GFR	
tubular function	

Renal elimination

There is an age-related decrease in creatinine clearance of 8mL/min/1.73m²/decade. Serum creatinine levels often remain within normal limits despite a decrease in GFR because the elderly generally have less muscle mass and thus produce less creatinine. Decreases in tubular function parallel those in glomerular function. These changes decrease renal elimination of some drugs. Creatinine clearance is used to guide drug dosing.

Pharmacodynamic changes with age

In the elderly, the effects of similar drug concentrations at the site of action may be greater or smaller than those in younger patients (see Table 8.3.2). Differences may be due to changes in:
- Drug-receptor interaction.
- Post-receptor events.
- Adaptive homeostatic responses.
- Pathological changes in organs.

Table 8.3.2 Examples of effect of ageing on drug response

Class	Drug	Action	Effect of Ageing
Analgesics	Morphine	Acute analgesic effect	↑
Anticoagulants	Warfarin	PT	↑
Bronchodilators	Salbutamol	Bronchodilation	↓
Cardiovascular drugs	Angiotensin II receptor blockers	Decreased blood pressure	↑
	Diltiazem	Acute antihypertensive effect	↑
	Enalapril	Acute antihypertensive effect	↑
	Verapamil	Acute antihypertensive effect, cardiac conduction effects	↑
Diuretics	Bumetanide	Increased urine flow and Na excretion	↓
	Furosemide	Latency and size of peak diuretic response	↓
Hypoglycaemics	Tolbutamide	Acute hypoglycaemic effect	↓
Psychoactive drugs	Diazepam	Sedation	↑
	Diphenhydramine	Psychomotor function	↑
	Haloperidol	Acute sedation	↑
	Midazolam	EEG activity	↑
	Temazepam	Postural sway	↑

Elderly patients are particularly sensitive to anticholinergic drug effects. Some drug categories (e.g. analgesics, anticoagulants, antihypertensives, anti-Parkinsonian drugs, diuretics, hypoglycaemic drugs, psychoactive drugs) pose special risks for elderly patients. Some, although reasonable for use in younger adults, are so risky as to be considered inappropriate for the elderly.

Further reading

Beers MH, Porter RS, Jones TV, Kaplan JL, Berkwits M, eds. (2006). *The Merck Manual of Diagnosis and Therapy*. 18th edn. NJ: Whitehouse Station.

Medicines for patients with hepatic impairment

Hepatic impairment

Metabolism of drugs occurs in two phases (see Fig. 8.4.1). Phase I, occurring mainly in the liver, consists of microsomal oxidation, reduction, and hydrolysis in the smooth endoplasmic reticulum and non-endoplasmic reticulum metabolism. Phase II metabolism consists of conjugation through either glucuronidation, amino acid conjugation, acetylation, methylation, sulphation, mercaptopuric acid formation, or glutathione conjugation.

Liver disease can therefore have multiple, often unpredictable effects on drug metabolism. AST, ALT, gamma-GT, and alkaline phosphatase all provide evidence of hepatocellular damage, but do not specifically indicate the ability of the liver to metabolize drugs. The best indicators of metabolic function for the liver are INR and serum albumin concentration as reflecting the ability of the liver to synthesize proteins. Serum albumin, however, is also reduced in other states, such as chronic malnutrition.

Where the definition of liver dysfunction is concerned, albumin<30g/L or INR>1.2 are the usual criteria.

Hepatic drug clearance

Hepatic drug clearance is a function of liver blood flow, and the intrinsic drug metabolizing capacity of the particular hepatic enzyme. The extraction ratio is the fraction of drug removed on one pass through the liver.

The elimination of high clearance drugs is determined by both hepatic blood flow and enzyme activity. The elimination of low clearance drugs is determined primarily by enzyme activity, as increased delivery of drug to the liver will not improve processing capacity.

Hepatic metabolism

Both phase I (P450-mediated metabolism) and phase II (conjugation) reactions are impacted by hepatic impairment. Overall, hepatic blood flow, intra-/extra-hepatic shunting of blood, and enzyme activity. Prediction of altered PK in hepatic impairment depends on knowledge about total drug clearance and hepatic extraction ratio.

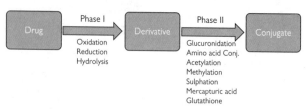

Fig. 8.4.1 The two phases of drug metabolism.

Specific liver disorders

Liver disorders known to decrease drug metabolism include:
- Cirrhosis.
- Alcoholic liver disease (chronic alcohol consumption is also recognized to induce enzymes responsible for drug metabolism, however).
- Viral hepatitis (may increase or decrease metabolism).
- Porphyria.

Cirrhosis, porphyria, and benign liver tumours do not appear to significantly alter hepatic glucuronidation and drugs solely eliminated via this mechanism are less likely to be affected (e.g. morphine, orazepam) than drugs that are not glucuronidated.

Management of drugs in liver disease

- Check the BNF/SmPC to determine route of metabolism if unsure.
- Calculate usual adult daily dose.
- For severe liver dysfunction (albumin < 30g/L, INR > 1.2) and high clearance drugs, reduce dose by 50%.
- For low clearance drugs, reduce dose by 25%.

Examples of high clearance drugs

- Antipsychotics.
- Beta-blockers (most).
- Calcium channel blockers.
- Lignocaine.
- Nitrates.
- Opioids (most).
- SSRIs.
- Statins.
- Tricyclic antidepressants.

Examples of low clearance drugs

- Amiodarone.
- Anticonvulsants (most).
- Antimalarials.
- Anti-Parkinsons (except amantadine).
- Antithyroid.
- Benzodiazepines.
- NSAIDs.
- Proton pump inhibitors.
- Paracetamol.
- Quinidine.
- Retinoids.
- Rifampicin.
- Spironolactone.
- Steroids.
- Sulphonylureas.
- Theophylline.
- Warfarin.

Low therapeutic index medications require extra caution. Where possible, switch to a drug that is renally eliminated or one that is conjugated, rather than oxidized via the P450 system.

Further reading

Canterbury District Health Board. Drug use in liver impairment. Available at: ℜ http://www.druginformation.co.nz/Bulletins/DrugsLiverDisease.pdf
BNF British National Formulary. Available at: ℜ http://bnf.org/bnf/bnf/current/204157.htm

Medicines for patients with renal impairment

Overview

The kidneys are involved to some degree in the elimination of virtually all drugs depending on the polarity of the drug or its metabolite. The kidneys manage drugs predominantly via 4 mechanisms:

- *Glomerular filtration*: filtering of free drug with MW < 66 000.
- *Proximal tubular secretion*: organic acids and bases (e.g. penicillin, sulphonamides, cimetedine).
- *Passive distal tubular reabsorption*:
  - Very lipophilic drugs mostly absorbed, e.g. griseofulvin.
  - Very polar drugs eliminated without reabsorption, e.g. mannitol.
  - High pH favours acid elimination and low pH favours base elimination.
- *Active tubular reabsorption*:
  - Minor role for most drugs.
  - For example, lithium.

Renal impairment can therefore have an important effect on drug pharmacokinetics and may therefore require adjustments.

Dose adjustment for impaired creatinine clearance

eGFR (estimated) bands are used as criteria for assessment of dose reduction in renal impairment. This is because the 5 stages of chronic kidney disease (CKD) are used in the stratification of patients entering a study:

- CKD 1 (>60mL/min) (normal or increased renal GFR, proteinuria).
- CKD 2 (>60mL/min) mildly decreased GFR.
- CKD 3 (30–59mL/min).
- CKD 4 (15–29mL/min).
- CKD 5 (<15mL/min).

Clear advice either for dose reduction or avoidance according to CKD band is given in the BNF. Examples of drugs that require dose reduction/avoidance in renal impairment include those that are highly water soluble, such as digoxin, or those that may exacerbate salt and water retention, such as NSAIDs.

Dose adjustment for decreased plasma proteins

Medicines that are highly protein bound may have significantly altered PK parameters in response to increased urinary protein excretion. Low serum albumin or reduced levels of other carrier proteins may therefore result in an increased fraction of free drug.

Examples of agents that are highly protein bound include warfarin and phenytoin; low plasma proteins therefore may be associated with an increase in INR or potentially increased toxicity from phenytoin due to an increase in free (unbound phenytoin).

A number of hormones are also bound to specific carrier proteins, which may be reduced when there is increased urinary protein excretion. Examples include thyroxine (bound to thyroid hormone-binding globulin) and sex steroids that are bound to sex hormone binding globulin.

Changes in protein binding associated with acute renal failure

Changes in free vs. bound drug may also occur in conditions of metabolic acidosis associated with renal failure. The prime example here is phenytoin, which under normal conditions is highly protein bound, and measured levels of phenytoin (incorporating both free and bound drug) are a valuable estimate of potential toxicity. Unfortunately, under conditions of renal impairment the proportion of free drug increases, and as such plasma levels of phenytoin become a very poor estimate of potential toxicity.

Assessment of new agents—organic anion transporters interactions

It is becoming increasingly apparent that drug interaction with renal organic anion transporters plays a potentially important role in nephrotoxicity of agents. These transporters not only play a role in drug excretion/resorption, but also potentially affect the excretion of metabolites such as uric acid. Those drugs which are particularly affected by OAT interaction are those which are more than 50% excreted by the kidney.

Examples of drugs that may be impacted by OAT interaction include antibiotics such as ciprofloxacin, certain antihistamines, pravastatin, and ACE inhibitors, such as ramipril and enalapril.

As such, assessment of potential OAT interaction is now an essential part of early clinical pharmacology studies.

Further reading

BNF. Available at: ℘ http://bnf.org/bnf/bnf/current/43768.htm

Chapter 8.6

Principles of benefit–risk

Benefit–risk

The assessment of benefit–risk is a complex multidimensional task, which requires the evaluation of all available and relevant data. Expert judgement is required, where data is translated into an overall conclusion about the balance between the perceived benefits and the perceived risks. Such an evaluation should take into account and compare the observed favourable effects, the observed unfavourable effects, as well as the uncertainties. Favourable effects are any known beneficial outcomes for the target population, unfavourable effects are any known detrimental outcomes and uncertainties arise from variation. The following points may be considered:

- Amount of evidence to characterize the benefit–risk.
- Availability of comparative data, the limitations of the data, and potential pitfalls of comparative analyses.
- Clinical relevance and context of the benefits and risks.
- Level of risk acceptability that corresponds to perceived degree of benefit in a specific context.
- How the benefit–risk may evolve over time.
- How the benefit–risk may vary across different factors and subgroups.
- Sensitivity of benefit risk balance to different assumptions.
- The perspective of different stakeholders regarding the risks, benefits and uncertainties.

Current research is exploring methodologies for benefit–risk analysis and assessment. These models include a range of quantitative and semi-quantitative tools that may assist in reaching a benefit–risk conclusion.

Benefit–risk in clinical development

There are a number of considerations regarding the use of human subjects in medical research. According to the World Medical Association Declaration of Helsinki's Ethical Principles for Medical Research Involving Human Subjects, the following apply:

- Every medical research study involving human subjects must be preceded by careful assessment of predictable risks and burdens to the individuals and communities involved in the research in comparison with foreseeable benefits to them and to other individuals or communities affected by the condition under investigation.
- Physicians may not participate in a research study involving human subjects unless they are confident that the risks involved have been adequately assessed and can be satisfactorily managed. Physicians must immediately stop a study when the risks are found to outweigh the potential benefits or when there is conclusive proof of positive and beneficial results.
- Medical research involving human subjects may only be conducted if the importance of the objective outweighs the inherent risks and burdens to the research subjects.

Benefit–risk assessment for a marketing authorization application

The assessment of the benefit–risk balance will be based on the available tests and studies submitted in an MAA. Under Community Law (Regulation 726/2004), authorization decisions should be taken on the basis of objective scientific criteria of quality, safety, and efficacy of the medicinal product concerned and Article 26 of Directive 2001/83/EC states that the MA shall be refused if the benefit–risk balance is not considered to be favourable or if therapeutic efficacy is insufficiently substantiated.

The benefit–risk assessment will determine the key benefits and harms and the strengths, uncertainties, and limitations of the data package. However, assessing the balance between the risks, benefits, and uncertainties of a NDA is a complex task and there are advantages to expressing the relationship between these factors in a formal framework. The European Medicines Agency's four-fold qualitative model of risk and benefits is one such framework, and it is illustrated in Table 8.6.1.

Table 8.6.1 European Medicines Agency model of risk and benefits

Favourable effects	Uncertainty of the favourable effects
Unfavourable effects	Uncertainty of the unfavourable effects

Reproduced with permission from The European Medicines Agency, 'Benefit Risk Methodology Project: Work package 1 report: description of the current practice of benefit-risk assessment for centralised procedure products in the EU regulatory network', Available at: ℘ http://www.ema.europa.eu/docs/en_GB/document_library/Report/2011/07/WC500109478.pdf © European Union, 1998–2012.

Further reading

EMA. Benefit–risk methodology. Available at: ℘ http://www.ema.europa.eu/ema/index.jsp?curl=pages/special_topics/document_listing/document_listing_000314.jsp&murl=menus/special_topics/special_topics.jsp&mid=WC0b01ac0580223ed6&jsenabled=true
World Medical Association Declaration of Helsinki. Ethical principles for medical research involving human subjects. Available at: ℘ http://www.wma.net/en/30publications/10policies/b3/17c.pdf

Therapeutic drug monitoring

Overview

Therapeutic drug monitoring is indicated for drugs that have a narrow therapeutic index; in other words, the dose range at which the agent is therapeutic is narrow vs. that above which significant side effects/adverse events of therapy occur.

For agents where PK monitoring is possible, and an effective dose range has been defined, this may take the form of assay of drug levels.

Where a predictable PD effect is known, this may take the form of assay of a PD marker associated with clinical effect.

Indications for PK drug monitoring include:
- There is an experimentally determined relationship between plasma drug concentration and the pharmacological effect.
- Knowledge of the drug level influences management.
- There is narrow therapeutic window.
- There are potential patient compliance problems.
- The drug dose cannot be optimized by observing changes in clinical parameters alone.

Examples of agents where PK assay is currently in clinical use

- *Gentamicin/aminoglycosides* (highly effective antibiotics, but toxic levels can result in permanent oto- or nephrotoxicity).
- *Anti-epileptics:* such as phenytoin or carbamazepine. (Note, however, that current phenytoin assays measure protein bound plus free phenytoin, free phenytoin levels increase significantly in renal impairment, which can result in toxicity symptoms in the normal range).
- *Lithium carbonate:* significant risk of chronic and acute toxicity at toxic plasma levels, with possible multiple adverse effects including renal impairment, and thyroid dysfunction.

Examples of agents where PD effects are monitored

- *Warfarin*: narrow therapeutic window between normal INR and INR at a level that risks significant bleeding.

Further reading

International Association of Therapeutic Drug Monitoring and Clinical Toxicology. Available at: http://www.iatdmct.org/

Index